S0-AWR-500

The Ministry *of* Health and Healing

An Adaptation of
The Ministry of Healing
by

Ellen G. White

Pacific Press® Publishing Association
Nampa, Idaho
Oshawa, Ontario, Canada
www.pacificpress.com

This book is dedicated to the Physicians, Nurses
and Medical Personnel of every land who, as co-workers with
the Chief Physician, the great Medical Missionary,
are selflessly ministering to the sick, comforting the afflicted,
and teaching the way of life.

Cover design by Eucaris L. Galicia

Copyright © 2004 by
The Ellen G. White® Estate, Inc.
Printed in United States of America
All rights reserved

Additional copies of this book are available by
calling toll free 1-800-765-6955 or by visiting
http://www.adventistbookcenter.com

Library of Congress Cataloging-in-Publication Data

White, Ellen Gould Harmon, 1827-1915.
The ministry of health and healing : Ellen White's classic work on
wellness in today's language : an adaptation of The ministry of healing
by Ellen G. White / Ellen G. White.
p. cm.
ISBN: 0-8163-2025-X
1. Health—Religious aspects—Seventh-day Adventists.
2. Medicine—Religious aspects—Seventh-day Adventists.
3. Seventh-day Adventists—Doctrines.
I.White, Ellen Gould Harmon, 1827-1915. Ministry of healing. II. Title

BR115.H4W55 2005
231.8'321—dc22   2004058744

04 05 06 07 08 · 5 4 3 2 1

Contents

Health Principles

The Home

The Essential Knowledge

The Worker's Need

Foreword

The world is sick. Wherever people live, suffering abounds. No wonder, then, that the search for relief from sickness and disease is intense!

It is not the Creator's purpose that members of the human family should be weighed down with a burden of pain, that their activities should be curtailed by illness, that their strength wane, and their life be cut short by disease. But all too frequently the laws established by God to govern life are violated, sin enters the heart, and people lose sight of their dependence upon God, the Source of life and health. Then follow the penalties of transgressing God's laws—pain, sickness, death.

God wants us to understand the laws that govern the body. He wants us to bring our life practices into harmony with those laws. This is a duty of prime importance. We need to understand the many factors that contribute to true happiness—a cheerful home, obedience to the laws of life, and proper relationships to other people.

When sickness comes, it is essential that we employ the varied agencies that, in cooperation with nature's efforts, will build up the body and restore health. There is also a larger and more important question—that of our relationship to the Creator who in the beginning gave life to human beings, who made every provision for their continued happiness, and who today is still deeply interested in their welfare.

In this volume, the author has brought within the reach of every man and woman, lay and professional, every father and mother, every boy and girl, a vast fund of helpful information on life and its laws, on obtaining health and keeping it, on disease and its remedies, on sin and the healing of the soul.

For one hundred years this book has provided instruction on how to acquire maximum physical and spiritual health, thus bringing hope to the despondent, cheer to the sick, and rest to the weary. It has been issued and reissued in many countries and has been translated into more than thirty of the world's leading languages.

The message and the truths set forth in the first edition one hundred years ago remain unchanged in the present volume. However, inasmuch as social customs and language styles have changed considerably during the past century, the present text is, in a sense, a twenty-first century "translation." Gender-inclusive language has been adopted, words with current meanings have been substituted for words that might be misunderstood or have little meaning today, and some sentence structures have been modernized. Unless otherwise noted, Scripture quotations are from the New King James Version (NKJV) of the Bible.

As the many new translations of the Bible have created a fresh interest in the Holy Scriptures, we believe that this edition, prepared in the offices of the White Estate at the request of the General Conference Health Ministries Department, will be warmly welcomed. We believe it will enable a new generation of readers to benefit physically and spiritually by its timeless, inspired message.

That this work, which sets forth a way of life that offers abounding health and involves unselfish service, may fully accomplish its mission is the sincere hope of the publishers and

The Trustees of the
Ellen G. White Estate

The True Medical Missionary

Chapter 1

Jesus, Our Example

Jesus came to this world as the unwearied servant of human need. He "'took our infirmities and bore our sicknesses'" that He might minister to every need of humanity. Matthew 8:17. He came to remove the burden of disease, wretchedness, and sin. It was His mission to bring complete restoration to men and women. He came to give them health, peace, and perfection of character.

Varied were the circumstances and needs of those who wanted His aid, and none who came to Him went away without receiving help. From Him flowed a stream of healing power, and in body, mind, and soul people were made whole.

The Savior's work was not restricted to any time or place. His compassion knew no limit. His work of healing and teaching was on so large a scale that there was no building in Palestine large enough to receive the multitudes that thronged to Him. His hospital was on the green hill slopes of Galilee, in the thoroughfares of travel, by the seashore, in the synagogues—in any place where the sick could be brought to Him. In every city, every town, every village through which He passed, He laid His hands upon the afflicted ones and healed them. Wherever there were hearts ready to receive His message, He comforted them with the assurance that their heavenly Father loved them. All day He ministered to those who came to Him, and in the evening He gave attention to those who worked through the day to earn a meager amount to support their families.

Jesus carried the awful weight of responsibility for the salvation of humanity. He knew that unless there was a decided change in the principles and purposes of the human race, all would be lost. This was the burden of His soul, and none could appreciate the weight that rested on Him. Through childhood, youth, and manhood He walked alone. Day by day He met trials and temptations; day by day He was brought into contact with evil and saw its power on those He was seeking to bless and save. Yet He did not become discouraged.

A Life of Self-sacrifice

Jesus gave first place to His mission, and all His wishes came second. He glorified His life by making everything in it subordinate to the will of His Father. When in His youth His mother found Him in the school of the rabbis and said, "'Son, why have You done this to us?'" He answered—and His answer is the keynote of His lifework—"'Why did you seek Me? Did you not know that I must be about My Father's business?'" Luke 2:48, 49.

His life was one of constant self-sacrifice. He had no home in this world except as the kindness of friends provided for Him as a wayfarer. He came to live in our behalf the life of the poorest and to walk and work among the needy and the suffering. Unrecognized and unhonored, He walked in and out among the people for whom He had done so much.

He was always patient and cheerful, and the afflicted hailed Him as a messenger of life and peace. He saw the needs of men and women, children and youth, and to all He gave the invitation, "Come to Me."

During His ministry, Jesus devoted more time to healing the sick than to preaching. His miracles testified to the truth of His statement that He came not to destroy but to save. Wherever He went, the tidings of His mercy preceded Him. Where He had passed, the objects of His compassion were rejoicing in health and trying out their newfound powers. Crowds were collecting around them to hear from their lips what the Lord had done. His voice was the first sound that many had ever heard. His name was the first word they had ever spoken. His face was the first they had ever looked upon. Why should they not love Jesus and praise Him! As He passed through the towns and cities He was like a vital current, spreading life and joy.

> "The people that sat in darkness
> Saw a great light,
> And to them that sat in the region and shadow of death,
> To them did light spring up."
> Matthew 4:16, ARV, margin.

The Savior made each work of healing an occasion for implanting divine principles in the mind and soul. This was the purpose of His work. He imparted earthly blessings to people that He might influence their hearts to receive the gospel of His grace.

Christ might have occupied the highest place among the teachers of the Jewish nation, but He preferred rather to take the gospel to the poor. He went from place to place that those in the highways and byways might hear the words of truth. By the sea, on the mountainside, in the streets of the city, in the synagogue, His voice was heard explaining the Scriptures. Often He taught in the outer court of the temple, that the Gentiles might hear His words.

The Prince of Teachers

So different were Christ's explanations of Scripture from those given by the scribes and Pharisees that the attention of the people was arrested. The rabbis dwelt on tradition, human theory, and speculation. Often that which men had written and taught about the Scripture was put in place of the Scripture itself. The subject of Christ's teaching was the Word of God. He answered questioners with a plain, "It is written," "What do the Scriptures say?" "How do you read?" Whenever an interest was awakened by either friend or foe, He presented the Word. With clearness and power He proclaimed the gospel message. His words shed a flood of light on the teachings of patriarchs and prophets, and the Scriptures came to the people as a new revelation. Never before had His hearers perceived in the Word of God such depth of meaning.

Never was there such an evangelist as Christ. Though He was the Majesty of heaven, He humbled Himself to take our nature, that He might meet men and women where they were. To all, rich and poor, free and bond, Christ, the Messenger of the covenant, brought the tidings of salvation. His fame as the Great Healer spread throughout Palestine. The sick came to places where He would pass, that they might call on Him for help. Others came eager to hear His words and hoping to be touched by His hand. Thus He went from city to city, from town to town, preaching the gospel and healing the sick— the King of glory clothed in the lowly garb of humanity.

He attended the great yearly festivals of the nation, and to the multitude absorbed in outward ceremony He spoke of heavenly things, bringing eternity within their view. To all He brought treasures from the storehouse of wisdom, speaking in simple language so that they could easily understand. By methods peculiarly His own, He helped all who were in sorrow or affliction. With tender, courteous grace He ministered to each sin-sick soul, bringing healing and strength.

As the Prince of teachers, Jesus presented truth in the context of people's own life experiences. Thus, being connected with sacred memories and emotions, the truth was unforgettable. He taught in a way that made the people feel that He identified fully with their interests and happiness. His instruction was so direct, His illustrations so appropriate, His words so sympathetic and cheerful, that His hearers were charmed. The simplicity and earnestness with which He addressed the needy made every word seem sacred.

Ministering to Both Poor and Rich

What a busy life Jesus led! Day by day He might be seen entering the humble homes of want and sorrow, speaking hope to the downcast and peace to the distressed. Gracious, tenderhearted, and full of pity, He went about lifting up the bowed-down and comforting the sorrowful. Wherever He went, He carried blessing.

While He ministered to the poor, Jesus also studied ways of reaching the rich. He made friends of the wealthy and cultured Pharisee, the Jewish nobleman, and the Roman ruler. He accepted their invitations, attended their feasts, and made Himself familiar with their interests and occupations, that He might gain access to their hearts and reveal to them the imperishable riches.

Christ came to this world to show that by receiving power from on high, human beings can lead lives unstained by sin. With unwearying patience and sympathetic helpfulness He met men and women in their necessities. By the gentle touch of grace He banished from the soul unrest and doubt, changing enmity to love and unbelief to confidence.

Jesus could say to whom He pleased, "Follow Me," and the one addressed arose and followed Him. The spell of the world's enchantment was broken. At the sound of His voice the spirit of greed and ambition fled from the heart, and the person arose, emancipated, to follow the Savior.

Christ recognized no distinction of nationality, rank, or creed. The scribes and Pharisees wanted their own nation and local community alone to benefit from the gifts of heaven, excluding the rest of God's family in the world. But Jesus came to break down every wall that separated people. He came to show that His gift of mercy and love is for everyone, like air, sunlight, or the showers of rain that refresh the earth.

The life of Jesus established a religion in which there is no caste, a religion by which Jew and Gentile, free and bond, are linked as members of one family, equal before God. His plans and actions were not influenced by political considerations. He made no difference between neighbors and strangers, friends and enemies. He was always looking for people who were thirsting for the waters of life.

He saw value in every human being and endeavored to apply the healing remedy to every soul. No matter what social environment He was in, He presented a lesson appropriate to the time and the circumstances. Every time He saw someone neglected or insulted, His heart was stirred to provide divine-human sympathy. He inspired with hope even the roughest and most unpromising people, assuring them that they might become blameless and harmless, attaining characters that would reveal that they were children of God.

Often Jesus met those who had drifted under Satan's control and felt unable to break from his power. To such people, discouraged, sick, tempted, fallen, He spoke words of tenderest pity, words that were needed and could be understood. Others He met who were fighting hard against the adversary of souls. These He encouraged to persevere, assuring them that they would win, for angels of God were on their side and would give them victory.

At the table of the publicans Jesus sat as an honored guest, by His sympathy and social kindliness showing that He recognized their dignity as humans, and they longed to become worthy of His confidence. Upon their thirsty hearts His words fell with blessed, life-giving power. New impulses were awakened, and these outcasts of society saw the possibility of a new life.

Though He was a Jew, Jesus mingled freely with the Samaritans, deliberately disregarding the Pharisaic customs and prejudices of His nation. He accepted the hospitality of this despised people, slept under their roofs, ate at their tables—partaking of the food prepared and served by their hands— taught in their streets, and treated them with the utmost kindness and courtesy. And while He drew their hearts to Him by the tie of human sympathy, His divine grace brought to them the salvation that the Jews rejected.

Personal Ministry

Christ neglected no opportunity to proclaim the gospel of salvation. Listen to His wonderful words to that one woman of Samaria who came to draw water as He was sitting by Jacob's well. "'Give Me a drink,'" He said, surprising her by asking a favor of her. He wanted some cool water, but He also wished to open a way by which He might give her the water of life. "'How is it,'" the woman asked, "'that You, being a Jew, ask a drink from me, a Samaritan woman?' For Jews have no dealings with Samaritans."

Jesus answered, "'If you knew the gift of God, and who it is who says to you, "Give Me a drink," you would have asked Him, and He would have given you living water. . . . Whoever drinks of this water will thirst again, but whoever drinks of the water that I shall give him will never thirst. But the water that I shall give him will become in him a fountain of water springing up into everlasting life.'" John 4:7-14.

How much interest Christ manifested in this one woman! How earnest and eloquent were His words! When the woman heard them, she left her water pot and went into the city, saying to her friends, "'Come, see a Man who told me all things that I ever did. Could this be the Christ?'" We read that "many of the Samaritans of that city believed in Him." Verses 29, 39. And who can estimate the influence that these words have had on the work of soul winning in the years that have passed since then?

Wherever hearts are open to receive the truth, Christ is ready to instruct them. He reveals to them the Father and the service acceptable to Him who reads the heart. For such, He uses no parables. To them, as to the woman at the well, He says, "I who speak to you am He."

Chapter 2

Days
of Ministry

In the fisherman's home at Capernaum, the mother of Peter's wife was lying sick of "a high fever," and "they told Him about her." Jesus "touched her hand, and the fever left her," and she arose and ministered to the Savior and His disciples. Luke 4:38; Mark 1:30; Matthew 8:15.

Rapidly the news spread. The miracle had been performed on the Sabbath, and for fear of the rabbis the people did not dare to come for healing until the sun had set. Then from the homes, the shops, the marketplaces, the inhabitants of the city pressed toward the humble dwelling that sheltered Jesus. The sick were brought on litters; they came leaning on staffs; or, supported by friends, they tottered feebly into the Savior's presence.

Hour after hour they came and went, for nobody knew whether tomorrow would find the Healer still among them. Never before had Capernaum witnessed a day like this. The air was filled with the voice of triumph and shouts of deliverance.

Not until the last sufferer had been relieved did Jesus cease His work. It was far into the night when the multitude scattered and silence settled down upon the home of Simon. The long, exciting day was past, and Jesus sought rest. But while the city was wrapped in slumber, the Savior, "having risen a long while before daylight, . . . went out and departed to a solitary place; and there He prayed." Mark 1:35.

Early in the morning Peter and his companions came to Jesus saying that already the people of Capernaum were looking for Him. With surprise they heard Christ's words, "'I must preach the kingdom of God to the other cities also, because for this purpose I have been sent.'" Luke 4:43.

In the excitement that then pervaded Capernaum, there was danger that the object of His mission would be lost sight of. Jesus was not satisfied to attract attention to Himself merely as a wonderworker or as a healer of physical disease. He was trying to draw people to Him as their Savior. They were eager to believe that He had come as a king to establish an earthly reign, but He wanted to turn their minds from the earthly to the spiritual. Mere worldly success would interfere with His work.

And the wonder of the careless crowd jarred upon His spirits. No self-assertion mingled with His life. The homage that the world gives to position, wealth, or talent was foreign to the Son of man. Jesus used none of the means that people employ to win allegiance or command homage. Centuries before His birth it had been prophesied of Him, "'He will not cry out, nor raise His voice, nor cause His voice to be heard in the street. A bruised reed He will not break, and the smoking flax He will not quench: He will bring forth justice for truth.'" Isaiah 42:2, 3.

The Pharisees tried to gain distinction by their exacting commitment to rituals, the showiness of their worship, and their charities. They thought to prove their devotion to religion by making it the theme of discussion. Disputes between opposing sects were loud and long, and it was not unusual to hear on the streets the voice of angry controversy from learned doctors of the law.

In marked contrast to all this was the life of Jesus. In His life there was no noisy disputation, no ostentatious worship, no act to gain applause. Christ was hid in God, and God was revealed in the character of His Son. To this revelation Jesus desired the minds of the people to be directed.

The Sun of Righteousness did not burst upon the world in splendor to dazzle the senses with His glory. It is written of Christ, "His going forth is established as the morning." Hosea 6:3. Quietly and gently the daylight breaks upon the earth, dispelling the darkness and waking the world to life. So did the Sun of Righteousness arise, "'with healing in His wings.'" Malachi 4:2.

"'Behold! My Servant whom I uphold,
My Elect One in whom My soul delights!'"
> Isaiah 42:1. (See also verses 5-7, 10-12.)

"'I will bring the blind by a way they did not know;
I will lead them in paths they have not known.
I will make darkness light before them,
And crooked places straight.
These things I will do for them, and not forsake them.'"
> Isaiah 42:16.

"Sing, O heavens, for the Lord has done it!
Shout, you lower parts of the earth;
Break forth into singing, you mountains,
O forest, and every tree in it!
For the LORD has redeemed Jacob,
And glorified Himself in Israel."
                    Isaiah 44:23.

From Herod's dungeon, John the Baptist watched and waited in disappointment and perplexity concerning the Savior's work. He sent two of his disciples to Jesus with the message: "'Are You the Coming One, or do we look for another?'" Matthew 11:3. The Savior did not answer the disciples' question at once. As they stood wondering at His silence, the afflicted were coming to Him. The voice of the Mighty Healer penetrated the deaf ear. A word, a touch of His hand, opened the blind eyes to see the light of day, the scenes of nature, the faces of friends, and the face of the Deliverer. His voice reached the ears of the dying, and they arose in health and vigor. Paralyzed demoniacs obeyed His word; their madness left them, and they worshiped Him. The poor peasants and laborers, who were shunned by the rabbis as unclean, gathered about Him, and He spoke to them the words of eternal life.

Thus the day wore away, the disciples of John seeing and hearing everything. At last Jesus called them to Him and told them to go and tell John what they had seen and heard. Then He added, "'Blessed is he who is not offended because of Me.'" Matthew 11:6.

The disciples took the message to John, and it was enough. He remembered the prophecy concerning the Messiah, "'The Lord has anointed Me to preach good tidings to the poor; He has sent Me to heal the brokenhearted, to proclaim liberty to the captives, and the opening of the prison to those who are bound; to proclaim the acceptable year of the Lord, and . . . to comfort all who mourn.'" Isaiah 61:1, 2. Jesus of Nazareth was the Promised One. The evidence of His divinity was seen in His ministry to the needs of suffering humanity. His glory was shown in His willingness to step down from His royal throne and be born into our low estate.

The Principles of Heaven

The works of Christ not only declared Him to be the Messiah, they showed in what manner His kingdom was to be established. To John was opened the same truth that had come to Elijah in the desert, when "a great and strong wind tore into the mountains and broke the rocks in pieces before the Lord, but the Lord was not in the wind; and after the wind an earthquake, but the Lord was not in the earthquake; and after the earthquake a fire, but the Lord was not in the fire; and after the fire" God spoke to the prophet by "a still small voice." 1 Kings 19:11, 12. So Jesus was to do His work, not by overturning thrones and kingdoms, not with pomp and outward display, but through speaking to human hearts by a life of mercy and self-sacrifice.

The kingdom of God comes not with outward show. It comes through the gentleness of the inspiration of His Word, through the inward working of His Spirit, the fellowship of the soul with Him who is its life. The greatest manifestation of its power is seen in human nature brought to the perfection of the character of Christ.

The followers of Christ are to be the light of the world, but God does not bid them make an effort to shine. He does not approve of any self-satisfied endeavor to display superior goodness. He desires that their souls shall be imbued with the principles of heaven; then, as they come into contact with the world, they will reveal the light that is in them. Their steadfast fidelity in every act of life will be a means of illumination.

Wealth or high position, costly equipment, architecture, or furnishings are not essential to the advancement of the work of God. Neither are achievements that win human applause and administer to vanity. Worldly display, however imposing, is of no value in God's sight. Above the seen and temporal, He values the unseen and eternal. The former is of worth only as it expresses the latter. The choicest productions of art possess no beauty that can compare with beauty of character, which is the fruit of the Holy Spirit's working in the soul.

When God gave His Son to our world, He endowed human beings with imperishable riches—riches compared with which all the treasured wealth of the world since it began is nothingness. Christ came to this world and stood before His earthly children with the hoarded love of eternity, and this is the treasure that, through our connection with Him, we are to receive, to reveal, and to impart.

Human effort will be efficient in the work of God just according to the consecrated devotion of the worker, who reveals the power of the grace of Christ to transform the life. We are to be distinguished from the world because God has placed His seal upon us, because He manifests in us His own character of love. Our Redeemer covers us with His righteousness.

In choosing men and women for His service, God does not ask whether they possess worldly wealth, learning, or eloquence. He asks, "Do they walk in such humility that I can teach them My way? Can I put My words into their lips? Will they represent Me?" God can use every person just in proportion as He can put His Spirit into the soul temple. The work that He will accept is the work that reflects His image. His followers are to bear, as their credentials to the world, the never-changing characteristics of His immortal principles.

Ministry to Mothers and Children

As Jesus ministered in the cities of ancient Israel, mothers with their sick and dying little ones in their arms pressed through the throng, seeking to come within reach of His notice. Behold these mothers, pale, weary, almost despairing, yet determined and persevering. Bearing their burden of suffering, they seek the Savior. As they are crowded back by the surging throng, Christ makes His way to them step by step until He is close by their side. Hope springs up in their hearts. Their tears of gladness fall as they catch His attention and look into the eyes expressing such pity and love.

Singling out one of the group, the Savior invites her confidence, saying, "What shall I do for you?" She sobs out her great want, "Master, that You would heal my child." Christ takes the little one from her arms, and disease flees at His touch. The pallor of death is gone; the life-giving current flows through the veins; the muscles receive strength. Words of comfort and peace are spoken to the mother. And then another case, just as urgent, is presented. Again Christ exercises His life-giving power, and all give praise and honor to Him who does wonderful things.

We dwell much on the greatness of Christ's life. We speak of the wonderful things that He accomplished, of the miracles that He performed. But His attention to things considered small is even higher proof of His greatness. Among the Jews it was customary for children to be brought to some rabbi that he might lay his hands on them in blessing, but the disciples thought the Savior's work too important to be interrupted in this way. When the mothers came wanting Him to bless their little ones, the disciples looked on them with disfavor. They thought these children too young to be benefited by a visit to Jesus and concluded that He would be displeased at their presence. But the Savior understood the care and burden of the mothers who were trying to train their children according to the Word of God. He had heard their prayers. He Himself had drawn them into His presence.

One mother with her child had left her home to find Jesus. On the way she told a neighbor her errand, and the neighbor wished to have Jesus bless her children. Thus several mothers came together with their little ones. Some of the children had passed beyond the years of infancy to childhood and youth. When the mothers explained what they wanted, Jesus heard with sympathy the timid, tearful request. But He waited to see how the disciples would treat them. When He saw the disciples reproving the mothers and sending them away, thinking to do Him a favor, He showed them their error, saying, "'Let the little children come to Me, and do not forbid them; for of such is the kingdom of God.'" Mark 10:14. He took the children in His arms, laid His hands on them, and gave them the blessings for which they came.

The mothers were comforted. They returned to their homes strengthened and blessed by the words of Christ. They were encouraged to take up their burdens with new cheerfulness and to work hopefully for their children.

Could the afterlife of that little group be opened before us, we would see the mothers recalling to the minds of their children the scene of that day and repeating to them the loving words of the Savior. We would see, too, how often, in after years, the memory of these words kept the children from straying from the "straight and narrow" path.

Christ is today the same compassionate Savior as when He walked upon earth. He is as truly the helper of mothers now as when He gathered the little ones to His arms in Judea. The children in our homes are as much the purchase of His blood as were the children of long ago.

Jesus knows the burden of every mother's heart. He who had a mother that struggled with poverty and privation sympathizes with every mother in her many cares. He who made a long journey in order to relieve the anxious heart of a Canaanite woman will do as much for the mothers of today. He who gave back to the widow of Nain her only son, and in His agony upon the cross remembered His own mother, is touched today by the mother's sorrow. In every grief and every need, He will comfort and help.

As mothers come to Jesus with their perplexities, they will find grace sufficient to aid them in the care of their children. The gates are open for every mother who would lay her burdens at the Savior's feet. He who said, "'Let the little children come to Me, and do not forbid them'" (Mark 10:14), still invites mothers to bring their little ones to be blessed by Him.

In the children who were brought to Jesus, He saw men and women who would be heirs of His grace and subjects of His kingdom. Some of them would become martyrs for His sake. He knew that these children would listen to Him and accept Him as their Redeemer far more readily than would adults, many of whom were worldly-wise and hardhearted. In teaching, Jesus came down to their level. He, the Majesty of heaven, answered their questions and simplified His important lessons to meet their childish understanding. He planted in their minds the seeds of truth that in after years would spring up and bear fruit unto eternal life.

When Jesus told the disciples not to forbid the children to come to Him, He was speaking to His followers in all ages—to officers of the church, ministers, helpers, and all Christians. Jesus is drawing the children, and He bids us, "Let them come," as if He would say, They will come if you do not hinder them. Let not your un-Christlike character misrepresent Jesus. Do not keep the little ones away from Him by your coldness and harshness. Never give them cause to feel that heaven would not be a pleasant place to them if you were there. Do not speak of religion as something that children cannot understand, or act as if they were not expected to accept Christ in their childhood. Do not give them the false impression that the religion of Christ is a religion of gloom, and that in coming to the Savior they must give up all that makes life joyful.

As the Holy Spirit moves upon the hearts of the children, cooperate with His work. Teach them that the Savior is calling them, that nothing can afford Him greater joy than for them to give themselves to Him in the bloom and freshness of their years.

The Savior regards with infinite tenderness the souls whom He has purchased with His blood. Because of His love, they are rightfully His. He looks upon them with unutterable longing. His heart is drawn out not only to the best-trained and most attractive children but to those who have objectionable traits of character by inheritance and through neglect. Many parents do not understand how much they are responsible for these traits in their children. They lack the tenderness and wisdom to deal with the erring ones whom they have made what they are. But Jesus looks upon these children with pity. He traces from cause to effect.

Christian workers may be Christ's agents in drawing these faulty and erring ones to the Savior. By wisdom and tact they may bind them to their hearts. They may give courage and hope, and through the grace of Christ may see these children transformed in character, so that it may be said of them, "Of such is the kingdom of God."

Five Small Barley Loaves Feed the Multitude

All day the people had crowded around Christ and His disciples as He taught beside the sea. They had listened to His gracious words, so simple and so plain that they were as the balm of Gilead to their souls. The healing of His divine hand had brought health to the sick and life to the dying. The day had seemed to them like heaven on earth, and they were unconscious of how long it had been since they had eaten anything.

The sun was sinking in the west, and yet the people lingered. Finally the disciples came to Christ, urging that for their own sake the multitude should be sent away. Many had come from far and had eaten nothing since morning. In the surrounding towns and villages they might be able to obtain food. But Jesus said, "'You give them something to eat.'" Matthew 14:16. Then, turning to Philip, He asked, "'Where shall we buy bread, that these may eat?'" John 6:5.

Philip looked over the sea of heads and thought how impossible it would be to provide food for so great a company. He answered that two hundred pennyworth [the wages of two hundred days' work] of bread would not be enough to divide among them so that each might have a little.

Jesus inquired how much food could be found among the company. "'There is a lad here,'" said Andrew, "'who has five barley loaves and two small fish, but what are they among so many?'" Verse 9. Jesus directed that these be brought to Him. Then He told the disciples to seat the people on the grass. When this was accomplished, He took the food and, "looking up to heaven, He blessed and broke and gave the loaves to the disciples; and the disciples gave to the multitudes. So they all ate and were filled, and they took up twelve baskets full of the fragments that remained." Matthew 14:19, 20.

It was by a miracle of divine power that Christ fed the multitude, yet how humble was the fare provided—only fish and barley loaves, which were the daily fare of the fisher-folk of Galilee.

Christ could have given the people a rich meal, but food prepared merely to gratify the appetite would have conveyed no lesson for their good. Through this miracle Christ desired to teach a lesson of simplicity. If people today were simple in their habits, living in harmony with nature's laws, as did Adam and Eve in the beginning, there would be an abundant supply for the needs of the human family. But selfishness and the indulgence of appetite have brought sin and misery, from excess on the one hand and from want on the other.

Jesus did not seek to attract the people to Him by gratifying the desire for luxury. To that great throng, weary and hungry after the long exciting day, the simple fare was an assurance both of His power and of His tender care for them in the common needs of life. The Savior has not promised His followers the luxuries of the world. They may even suffer poverty, but His word is pledged that their need shall be supplied. He has promised that which is better than earthly good—the abiding comfort of His own presence.

After the multitude had been fed, there was an abundance of food left. Jesus told His disciples, "'Gather up the fragments that remain, so that nothing is lost.'" John 6:12. These words meant more than putting the food into baskets. The lesson was twofold. Nothing is to be wasted. We are to prize every temporal advantage. We should neglect nothing that would serve to benefit a human being. Let everything be gathered up that will relieve the necessities of earth's hungry ones. With the same carefulness we are to treasure the bread from heaven to satisfy the needs of the soul. By every word of God we are to live. Nothing that God has spoken is to be lost. Not one word that concerns our eternal salvation are we to neglect. Not one word is to fall useless to the ground.

The miracle of the loaves teaches dependence upon God. When Christ fed the five thousand, food was not close at hand. Apparently He had no funds to draw on. There He was, with five thousand men, besides women and children, in the wilderness. He had not invited the multitude to follow Him to this place. Eager to be in His presence, they had come without invitation or command; but He knew that after listening all day to His instruction they were hungry and faint. They were far from home, and the night was at hand. Many of them were without money to purchase food. He who for their sake had fasted forty days in the wilderness would not consent for them to return fasting to their homes.

The providence of God had placed Jesus where He was, and He depended on His heavenly Father for means to meet the emergency. When we are brought into crisis situations, we are to depend on God. In every emergency we are to seek help from Him who has infinite resources at His command.

In this miracle, Christ received from the Father and imparted to the disciples. The disciples imparted to the people, and the people to one another. So all who are united to Christ will receive from Him the bread of life and impart it to others. His disciples are the appointed means of communication between Christ and the people.

When the disciples heard the Savior's direction, "'You give them something to eat,'" all the difficulties arose in their minds. They questioned, "'Shall we go into the villages to buy food?'" But what did Christ say? "'*You* give them something to eat.'" The disciples brought to Jesus all they had, but He did not invite them to eat. He told them to serve the people. The food multiplied in His hands, and the hands of the disciples, reaching out to Christ, were never empty. The little supply available was sufficient for all. When the multitude had been fed, the disciples ate with Jesus of the precious, heaven-supplied food.

As we see the needs of the poor, the ignorant, the afflicted, how often our hearts sink. We question, "What can our feeble strength and slender resources do to supply this terrible necessity? Shall we not wait for someone of greater ability to direct the work, or for some organization to undertake it?" Christ says, "*You* give them something to eat." Use the means, the time, the ability, you have. Bring your barley loaves to Jesus.

Though your resources may not be sufficient to feed thousands, they may suffice to feed one. In the hand of Christ they may feed many. Like the disciples, give what you have. Christ will multiply the gift. He will reward honest, simple reliance upon Him. That which seemed but a meager supply will prove to be a rich feast.

"He who sows sparingly will also reap sparingly, and he who sows bountifully will also reap bountifully. . . . God is able to make all grace abound toward you, that you, always having all sufficiency in all things, have an abundance for every good work. As it is written:

'He has dispersed abroad,
He has given to the poor;
His righteousness endures forever.'

"Now may He who supplies seed to the sower, and bread for food, supply and multiply the seed you have sown and increase the fruits of your righteousness, while you are enriched in everything for all liberality." 2 Corinthians 9:6-11.

Chapter 3

With Nature
and With God

The Savior's life on earth was a life of communion with nature and with God. In this communion He revealed for us the secret of a life of power.

Jesus was an earnest, constant worker. No other person was ever so weighted with responsibilities. Never another carried so heavy a burden of the world's sorrow and sin. Never another worked with such self-consuming zeal for the good of humanity. Yet His was a life of health. Physically as well as spiritually He was represented by the sacrificial lamb, "without blemish and without spot." 1 Peter 1:19. In body and in soul He was an example of what God designed all humanity to be through obedience to His laws.

As the people looked upon Jesus, they saw a face in which divine compassion was blended with conscious power. He seemed to be surrounded with an atmosphere of spiritual life. Though His manners were gentle and unassuming, He impressed people with a sense of power that was hidden yet could not be wholly concealed.

During His ministry He was continually pursued by crafty and hypocritical men who were seeking His life. Spies were on His track, watching His words to find some occasion against Him. The keenest and most highly cultured minds of the nation tried to defeat Him in controversy. But never could they gain an advantage. They had to withdraw from the field, confounded and put to shame by the lowly Teacher from Galilee. Christ's teaching had a freshness and a power such as mortals had never before known.

Even His enemies were forced to confess, "'No man ever spoke like this Man!'" John 7:46.

The childhood of Jesus, spent in poverty, had been uncorrupted by the artificial habits of a corrupt age. Working at the carpenter's bench, bearing the burdens of home life, learning the lessons of obedience and toil, He found recreation amidst the scenes of nature, gathering knowledge as He sought to understand nature's mysteries. He studied the Word of God, and His hours of greatest happiness were found when He could leave the scene of His labors to go into the fields, to meditate in the quiet valleys, and hold communion with God on the mountainside or amid the trees of the forest. The early morning often found Him in some secluded place, meditating, searching the Scriptures, or praying. With the voice of singing He welcomed the morning light. With songs of thanksgiving He cheered His hours of work and brought heaven's gladness to the toil-worn and disheartened.

During His ministry, to a great degree Jesus lived an outdoor life. His journeys from place to place were made on foot, and much of His teaching was given in the open air. In training His disciples He often withdrew from the confusion of the city to the quiet of the fields, as more in harmony with the lessons of simplicity, faith, and self-abnegation He desired to teach them. It was beneath the sheltering trees of the mountainside, only a little distance from the Sea of Galilee, that He called the Twelve to the apostolate and gave the Sermon on the Mount.

Christ loved to gather the people about Him under the blue heavens, on a grassy hillside, or on a beach beside the lake. Here, surrounded by the works of His own creation, He could turn their thoughts from the artificial to the natural. In the growth and development of nature were revealed the principles of His kingdom. As the people lifted their eyes to the hills of God and saw the wonderful works of His hand, they learned precious lessons of divine truth. In the future the lessons of the divine Teacher would thus be repeated to them by the things of nature. The mind would be uplifted and the heart would find rest.

Jesus often released His disciples for a season, that they might visit their homes and rest; but they never succeeded in drawing Him away from His labors. All day He ministered to the throngs that came to Him, and at eventide, or in the early morning, He went away to the sanctuary of the mountains for communion with His Father.

Often His incessant labor and the conflict with the enmity and false teaching of the rabbis left Him so utterly wearied that His mother and brothers, and even His disciples, feared that His life would be sacrificed. But as He returned from the hours of prayer that closed the toilsome day, they noted the look of peace on His face, and the freshness, life, and power that seemed to pervade His whole being. From hours spent alone with God He came forth, morning by morning, to bring the light of heaven to the world.

Renewing Spiritual Energy

Just after returning from their first missionary tour Jesus invited His disciples to "'Come aside . . . and rest a while.'" The disciples had returned, filled with the joy of their success as heralds of the gospel, when the tidings reached them of the death of John the Baptist at the hand of Herod. It was a bitter sorrow and disappointment. Jesus knew that in leaving the Baptist to die in prison He had severely tested the disciples' faith. With pitying tenderness He looked upon their sorrowful, tear-stained faces. Tears were in His own eyes and voice as He said, "'Come aside by yourselves to a deserted place and rest a while.'" Mark 6:31.

Near Bethsaida, at the northern end of the Sea of Galilee, was a lonely region, beautiful with the fresh green of spring, that offered a welcome retreat to Jesus and His disciples. For this place they set out, going in their boat across the lake. Here they could rest, away from the confusion of the multitude. Here the disciples could listen to the words of Christ, undisturbed by the retorts and accusations of the Pharisees. Here they hoped to enjoy a short season of fellowship with their Lord.

Jesus had only a short time alone with His beloved ones, but how precious to them were those few moments. They talked together regarding the work of the gospel and the possibility of making their efforts more effective in reaching the people. As Jesus opened to them the treasures of truth, they were vitalized by divine power and inspired with hope and courage.

But soon the multitude was again looking for Him. Supposing that He had gone to His usual place of retirement, the people followed Him there. His hope to gain even one hour of rest was frustrated. But in the depth of His pure, compassionate heart the Good Shepherd of the sheep had only love and pity for these restless, thirsting souls. All day He ministered to their needs, and at evening dismissed them to go to their homes and rest.

In a life wholly devoted to the good of others, the Savior found it necessary to turn aside from ceaseless activity and contact with human needs, to seek retirement and unbroken communion with His Father. As the throng that had followed Him departed, He went into the mountains, and there, alone with God, poured out His soul in prayer for these suffering, sinful, needy ones.

When Jesus said to His disciples that the harvest was great and the workers were few, He did not urge upon them the necessity of ceaseless toil, but counseled them, "'Ask the Lord of the harvest to send out laborers into his harvest.'" Matthew 9:38, NRSV. To His toilworn workers today as really as to His first disciples He speaks these words of compassion, "Come aside by yourselves . . . and rest a while."

All who are under the training of God need the quiet hour for communion with their own hearts, with nature, and with God. In them is to be revealed a life that is not in harmony with the world, its customs, or its practices, and they need to have a personal experience in obtaining a knowledge of the will of God. We must individually hear Him speaking to the heart. When every other voice is hushed, and in quietness we wait before Him, the silence of the soul makes more distinct the voice of God. He bids us, "Be still, and know that I am God." Psalm 46:10.

This is the effectual preparation for all service for God. Amidst the hurrying throng and the strain of life's intense activities, all who are thus refreshed will be surrounded with an atmosphere of light and peace. They will receive a new endowment of both physical and mental strength. Their lives will breathe out a fragrance and will reveal a divine power that will reach people's hearts.

Chapter 4

The Touch
of Faith

"'If only I may touch His garment, I shall be made well.'" Matthew 9:21. A poor woman spoke these words, a woman who for twelve years had suffered from a disease that made her life a burden. She had spent all her money on physicians and remedies, only to be pronounced incurable. But as she heard of the Great Healer, her hopes revived. She thought, "If only I could get near enough to speak to Him, I might be healed."

Christ was on His way to the home of Jairus, the Jewish rabbi who had pleaded with Him to come and heal his daughter: "'My little daughter lies at the point of death. Come and lay Your hands on her, that she may be healed'" (Mark 5:23). Jairus's heartbroken petition had touched the tender, sympathetic heart of Christ. At once He set out with the ruler for his home.

They made slow progress, for the crowd pressed Christ on every side. Finally, the Savior came near to where the afflicted woman was standing. Again and again she had tried in vain to get near Him. Now her opportunity had come. She could see no way of speaking to Him. She would not try to hinder His slow advance. But she had heard that healing came from a touch of His garments, and, fearful of losing her one chance for relief, she pressed forward, saying to herself, "'If only I may touch His garment, I shall be made well.'"

Christ knew every thought of her mind, and He was making His way to where she stood. He realized her great need, and He was helping her to exercise faith.

As He was passing, she reached forward and succeeded in barely touching the border of His garment. That moment she knew that she was healed.

In that one touch was concentrated the faith of her life, and instantly her pain and feebleness disappeared. She felt the thrill as of an electric current passing through her body, restoring her to perfect health. "She felt in her body that she was healed of the affliction." Verse 29.

The grateful woman desired to thank the Mighty Healer who had done more for her in one touch than the physicians had done in twelve long years, but she dared not. With a grateful heart she tried to withdraw from the crowd. Suddenly Jesus stopped, then, looking around, asked, "Who touched Me?"

Looking at Him in amazement, Peter answered, "'Master, the multitudes throng You and press You, and You say, "Who touched Me?"'" Luke 8:45.

"'Somebody touched Me,'" Jesus said, "'for I perceived power going out from Me.'" Verse 46. He could distinguish the touch of faith from the casual touch of the careless crowd. Someone had touched Him with a deep purpose and had received an answer.

Christ had not asked the question for His own information. He had a lesson for the people, for His disciples, and for the woman. He wished to inspire the afflicted with hope and to show that it was faith that had brought the healing power. The woman's trust must not be passed by without comment. God must be glorified by the woman's grateful confession. Christ desired her to understand that He approved her act of faith. He would not have her leave with a half blessing only. She must not remain ignorant of His compassionate love and of His approval of her faith in His power to save to the uttermost all who come to Him.

Looking toward the woman, Christ insisted on knowing who had touched Him. Finding concealment impossible, she came forward trembling, and cast herself at His feet. With grateful tears, before all the people she told Him why she had touched His garment and how she had been healed immediately. She feared that it had been presumptuous of her to touch His garment, but no word of censure came from Christ's lips. He spoke only words of approval. They came from a heart of love, filled with sympathy for human woe. "'Daughter,'" He said gently, "'be of good cheer; your faith has made you well. Go in peace.'" Verse 48. How happy these words made her! Now no fear that she had offended Jesus embittered her joy.

To the curious crowd pressing about Jesus no vital power was imparted. But the suffering woman who touched Him in faith received healing. So in spiritual things the casual contact differs from the touch of faith. To believe in Christ merely as the Savior of the world can never bring healing to the soul. The faith that brings salvation is not a mere assent to the truth of the gospel. True faith is that which receives Christ as a personal Savior. God gave His only-begotten Son, that *I*, by believing in Him, "should not perish but have everlasting life." John 3:16. When I come to Christ, according to His word I am to believe that I receive His saving grace. The life that I now live, I am to "live by faith in the Son of God, who loved *me* and gave Himself for *me*." See Galatians 2:20.

Many hold faith as an opinion. Saving faith is a transaction, by which those who receive Christ join themselves in covenant relation with God. A living faith means an increase of vigor, a confiding trust, by which, through the grace of Christ, the soul becomes a conquering power.

Faith is a mightier conqueror than death. If the sick can be led to fix their eyes in faith upon the Mighty Healer, we shall see wonderful results. It will bring life to both body and soul.

In working for the victims of evil habits, instead of pointing them to the despair and ruin toward which they are hastening, turn their eyes away to Jesus. Fix them upon the glories of heavenly things. This will do more for saving both body and soul than will all the terrors of the grave when kept before the helpless and apparently hopeless.

A Centurion's Servant Healed

A centurion's servant was lying sick with palsy. Among the Romans the servants were slaves, bought and sold in the marketplaces, and often were treated with abuse and cruelty. But the centurion was tenderly attached to his servant and greatly desired to have him recover. He believed that Jesus could heal him. He had not seen the Savior, but the reports he had heard inspired him with faith. Despite the formalism of the Jews, this Roman was convinced that their religion was superior to his own. Already he had broken through the barriers of national prejudice and hatred that separated the conquerors from the conquered people. He had manifested respect for the service of God and had shown kindness to the Jews as His worshipers. In the teaching of Christ, as it had been reported to him, he found that which met the need of the soul. All that was spiritual within him responded to the Savior's words. But feeling himself unworthy to approach Jesus, he appealed to the Jewish elders to ask that his servant be healed.

The elders present the case to Jesus, urging that "the one for whom He should do this was deserving, 'for he loves our nation, and has built us a synagogue.'" Luke 7:4, 5.

But on the way to the centurion's home, Jesus receives a message from the officer himself, "'Lord, do not trouble Yourself, for I am not worthy that You should enter under my roof.'" Verse 6.

Still the Savior keeps on His way, and the centurion comes in person to complete the message, saying, "'Therefore I did not even think myself worthy to come to You. But say the word, and my servant will be healed. For I also am a man placed under authority, having soldiers under me. And I say to this one, "Go," and he goes; and to another, "Come," and he comes; and to my servant, "Do this," and he does it.'" Verses 7, 8.

"I represent the power of Rome, and my soldiers recognize my authority as supreme. So do You represent the power of the infinite God, and all created things obey Your word. You can command the disease to depart, and it shall obey You. Just say the word, and my servant will be healed."

"'As you have believed,'" Christ said, "'let it be done for you.' And his servant was healed that same hour." Matthew 8:13.

The Jewish elders had commended the centurion to Christ because of the favor he had shown to "'our nation.'" He is worthy, they said, for he "'has built us a synagogue.'" But the centurion said of himself, "'I am not worthy.'" Yet he did not fear to ask help from Jesus. Not to his own goodness did he trust, but to the Savior's mercy. His only argument was his great need.

In the same way every human being can come to Christ. "Not by works of righteousness which we have done, but according to His mercy He saved us." Titus 3:5. Do you feel that because you are a sinner you cannot hope to receive blessing from God? Remember that Christ came into the world to save sinners. We have nothing to recommend us to God; the plea that we may urge now and always is our utterly helpless condition, which makes His redeeming power a necessity. Renouncing all self-dependence, we may look to the cross of Calvary and say:

"In my hand no price I bring;
Simply to Thy cross I cling."

"'If you can believe, all things are possible to him who believes.'" Mark 9:23. It is faith that connects us with heaven and brings us strength for coping with the powers of darkness. In Christ, God has provided means for subduing every evil trait and resisting every temptation, however strong. Many feel that they lack faith, therefore they remain away from Christ. But these souls, in their helpless unworthiness, should cast themselves upon the mercy of their compassionate Savior. Don't look to self but to Christ. He who healed the sick and cast out demons when He was on earth is still the mighty Redeemer. Then grasp His promises as leaves from the tree of life: "'The one who comes to Me I will by no means cast out.'" John 6:37. As you come to Him, believe that He accepts you, because He has promised. You can never perish while you do this—never.

"God demonstrates His own love toward us, in that while we were still sinners, Christ died for us." Romans 5:8. And "if God is for us, who can be against us? He who did not spare His own Son, but delivered Him up for us all, how shall He not with Him also freely give us all things?" Romans 8:31, 32.

"I am persuaded that neither death nor life, nor angels nor principalities nor powers, nor things present nor things to come, nor height nor depth, nor any other created thing, shall be able to separate us from the love of God which is in Christ Jesus our Lord." Verses 38, 39.

A Leper Is Cleansed

Of all the diseases known in the East, leprosy was most dreaded. Its incurable, contagious character, and its horrible effect on its victims, filled the bravest with fear. Among the Jews it was regarded as a judgment on account of sin, and hence was called "the stroke," "the finger of God." Deep-rooted, ineradicable, deadly, it was looked upon as a symbol of sin.

By ritual law the leper was pronounced unclean. Whatever he touched was unclean. The air was polluted by his breath. Like one already dead, he was shut out from society and home. One who was suspected of having the disease must present himself to the priests, who were to examine and decide his case. If pronounced a leper, he was isolated from his family, cut off from the congregation of Israel, and doomed to associate only with those who were similarly afflicted. Even kings and rulers were not exempt. A monarch attacked by this terrible disease must yield his throne and flee from society.

Away from friends and kindred, the leper must bear the curse of his malady. He was obliged to declare his condition, rend his clothes, and sound the alarm, warning all to flee from his contaminating presence. The cry "Unclean! unclean!" coming in mournful tones from the lonely exile, was a signal heard with fear and abhorrence.

In the region of Christ's ministry were many of these sufferers, and as the news of His work reaches them, faith begins to spring up in the heart of one man. If he could go to Jesus, he might be healed. But how can he find Jesus? Doomed as he is to perpetual isolation, how can he present himself to the Healer? And will Christ heal him? Will He not, like the Pharisees, and even the physicians, pronounce a curse on him and warn him to keep away from places where people congregate?

He thinks of all he has been told of Jesus. Not a single person who has asked His help has been turned away. The wretched man determines to find the Savior. Though forbidden to enter the cities, it may be that he can cross the Healer's path on some mountain trail or find Him as He is teaching outside the towns. The difficulties are great, but this is his only hope.

Standing afar off, the leper catches a few words from the Savior's lips. He sees Him laying His hands on the sick. He sees the lame, the blind, the paralytic, and those dying of various maladies rise up in health, praising God for deliverance. His faith strengthens. Nearer and yet nearer he approaches the listening crowd. The restrictions laid upon him, the safety of the people, and the fear with which everyone regards him—all are forgotten. He thinks only of the blessed hope of healing.

He is a loathsome spectacle. His decaying body is repulsive. At sight of him the people fall back. In their terror they crowd upon one another to escape from contact with him. Some try to prevent him from approaching Jesus, but in vain. He neither sees nor hears them. He sees only the Son of God, he hears only the voice that speaks life to the dying.

Pressing to Jesus, he casts himself at His feet with the cry, "'Lord, if You are willing, You can make me clean.'"

Jesus replies, "'I am willing; be cleansed,'" and lays His hand upon him. Matthew 8:2, 3.

Immediately a change passes over the leper. His blood becomes healthy, the nerves sensitive, the muscles firm. The unnaturally white, scaly surface peculiar to leprosy disappears, and his flesh becomes as the flesh of a little child.

If the priests were to learn the facts concerning the healing of the leper, their hatred of Christ might lead them to render a dishonest sentence. Jesus desired that an impartial decision be secured. He therefore advised the man to tell no one of the cure but without delay present himself at the temple with an offering before rumors concerning the miracle are spread abroad. Before the priests could accept such an offering, they were required to examine the offerer and certify his complete recovery.

This examination was made. The priests who earlier had condemned the leper to banishment testified to his cure. The healed man was restored to his home and society. He rejoiced in the vigor of manhood and in being restored to his family.

Notwithstanding the caution of Jesus, the man could no longer conceal the fact of his cure, and joyfully he went about proclaiming the power of the One who had made him whole.

When this man came to Jesus, he was "full of leprosy." Its deadly poison permeated his whole body. The disciples tried to prevent their Master from touching him, for anyone who touched a leper became unclean. But in laying His hand on the leper, Jesus received no defilement. The leprosy was cleansed. Thus it is with the leprosy of sin—deep-rooted, deadly, impossible to be cleansed by human power. "The whole head is sick, and the whole heart faints. From the sole of the foot even to the head, there is no soundness in it, but wounds and bruises and putrefying sores." Isaiah 1:5, 6. But Jesus, coming to dwell in humanity, receives no pollution. His presence provides healing virtue for the sinner. Whoever will fall at His feet, saying in faith, "Lord, if You are willing, You can make me clean," shall hear the answer, "I am willing. Be cleansed."

In some instances, Jesus did not at once grant healing. But in the case of leprosy, no sooner was the appeal made than it was granted. When we pray for earthly blessings, the answer to our prayer may be delayed, or God may give us something other than what we ask for. But not so when we ask for deliverance from sin. It is His will to cleanse us from sin, to make us His children, and to enable us to live a holy life. Christ "gave Himself for our sins, that He might deliver us from this present evil age, according to the will of our God and Father." Galatians 1:4. "Now this is the confidence that we have in Him, that if we ask anything according to His will, He hears us. And if we know that He hears us, whatever we ask, we know that we have the petitions that we have asked of Him." 1 John 5:14, 15.

Jesus looked on the distressed and heart-burdened, those whose hopes were disappointed, and who with earthly joys were seeking to quiet the longing of the soul, and He invited all to find rest in Him.

"You Will Find Rest"

Tenderly He urged the toiling people, "'Take My yoke upon you and learn from Me, for I am gentle and lowly in heart, and you will find rest for your souls.'" Matthew 11:29.

In these words, Christ was speaking to every human being. Whether they know it or not, all are weary and heavy-laden. All are weighed down with burdens that only Christ can remove. The heaviest burden that we bear is the burden of sin. If we were left to bear this burden, it would crush us. But the Sinless One has taken our place. "The Lord has laid on Him the iniquity of us all." Isaiah 53:6.

He has borne the burden of our guilt. He will take the load from our weary shoulders. He will give us rest. The burden of care and sorrow also He will bear. He invites us to cast all our care upon Him, for He carries us upon His heart.

The Elder Brother of our race is by the eternal throne. He sees every soul who is looking toward Him as the Savior. He knows by experience what are the weaknesses of humanity, what are our wants, and where lies the strength of our temptations, for He was "in all points tempted as we are, yet without sin." Hebrews 4:15. He is watching over you, trembling child of God. Are you tempted? He will deliver. Are you weak? He will strengthen. Are you ignorant? He will enlighten. Are you wounded? He will heal. The Lord "counts the number of the stars," and yet "He heals the brokenhearted and binds up their wounds." Psalm 147:4, 3.

Whatever your anxieties and trials, lay your case before the Lord. Your spirit will be braced for endurance. The way will be open for you to disentangle yourself from embarrassment and difficulty. The weaker and more helpless you know yourself to be, the stronger will you become in His strength. The heavier your burdens, the more blessed the rest in casting them upon your Burden Bearer.

Circumstances may separate friends; the restless waters of the wide sea may roll between us and them. But no circumstances, no distance, can separate us from the Savior. Wherever we may be, He is at our right hand to support, maintain, uphold, and cheer. Christ's love for His redeemed is greater than the love of a mother for her child. It is our privilege to rest in His love, to say, "I will trust Him, for He gave His life for me."

Human love may change, but Christ's love never changes. When we cry to Him for help, His hand is stretched out to save.

"'The mountains shall depart
And the hills be removed,
But My kindness shall not depart from you,
Nor shall My covenant of peace be removed,'
Says the Lord, who has mercy on you."
Isaiah 54:10.

Chapter 5

Healing of the Soul

Many of those who came to Christ for help had brought disease on themselves, yet He did not refuse to heal them. And when virtue from Him entered into these people, they were convicted of sin. Many were healed of their spiritual disease as well as of their physical maladies.

Among these was the paralytic at Capernaum. Like the leper, this man had lost all hope of recovery. His disease was the result of a sinful life, and his sufferings were embittered by remorse. He had appealed to the Pharisees and physicians for relief, but they pronounced him incurable. They denounced him as a sinner and declared that he would die under the wrath of God.

The palsied man had sunk into despair. Then he heard of Jesus. Others, as sinful and helpless as he, had been healed, and he was encouraged to believe that he, too, might be cured if he could be carried to the Savior. But hope fell as he remembered the cause of his malady. Yet he could not dismiss the possibility of healing.

His great desire was relief from the burden of sin. He longed to see Jesus and receive the assurance of forgiveness and peace with heaven. Then he would be content to live or die, according to God's will.

There was no time to lose. Already his wasted flesh bore signs of death. He asked his friends to carry him on his bed to Jesus, and this they gladly set out to do. But so dense was the crowd that had assembled in and around the house where the Savior was that it was impossible for the sick man and his friends to reach Him. They were unable to get close enough even to hear His voice.

Jesus was teaching in the home of Peter. As usual, His disciples sat close to Him, and "there were Pharisees and teachers of the law sitting by, who had come out of every town of Galilee, Judea, and Jerusalem." Luke 5:17. Many of these had come as spies, looking for reasons to criticize Jesus. Beyond these thronged a mixed multitude—the eager, the reverent, the curious, and the unbelieving. Different nationalities and all levels of society were represented. "And the power of the Lord was present to heal." Verse 17. The Spirit of life brooded over the assembly, but the Pharisees and lawyers did not discern His presence. They felt no sense of need, and the healing was not for them. "He has filled the hungry with good things, and the rich He has sent away empty." Luke 1:53.

Again and again the men bearing the paralytic tried to push their way through the crowd, but failed. The sick man looked about him in unutterable anguish. How could he relinquish hope when the longed-for help was so near? At his suggestion his friends carried him to the top of the house, then broke up the roof and let him down at the feet of Jesus.

The Savior looked upon the mournful countenance and saw the pleading eyes fixed upon Him. He well knew the longing of that burdened soul. It was He who had brought conviction to his conscience when he was yet at home. When he repented of his sins and believed in the power of Jesus to make him whole, the mercy of the Savior had blessed his heart. Jesus had watched the first glimmer of faith grow into a conviction that He was the sinner's only helper, and had seen it grow stronger with every effort to come into His presence. It was Christ who had drawn the sufferer to Himself. Now, in words that fell like music on the listener's ear, the Savior said, "'Son, be of good cheer; your sins are forgiven you.'" Matthew 9:2.

The burden of guilt rolls from the sick man's soul. He cannot doubt. Christ's words reveal His power to read the heart. Who can deny His power to forgive sins? Hope takes the place of despair, and joy replaces oppressive gloom. The man's physical pain is gone, and his whole being is transformed. Making no further request, he lay in peaceful silence, too happy for words.

Many were watching with breathless interest every movement in this strange transaction. Many felt that Christ's words were an invitation to them. Were they not soul-sick because of sin? Did they not want to be free from this burden?

But the Pharisees, fearful of losing their influence with the multitude, said in their hearts, "'Why does this Man speak blasphemies like this? Who can forgive sins but God alone?'" Mark 2:7.

Jesus fixed His glance upon them, and as they cowered and drew back He said, "'Why do you think evil in your hearts? For which is easier, to say, "Your sins are forgiven you," or to say, "Arise and walk"? But that you may know that the Son of Man has power on earth to forgive sins,'" He said,

turning to the paralytic, "'Arise, take up your bed, and go to your house.'"
Matthew 9:4-6.

Then the paralytic who had been carried on a litter to Jesus rose to
his feet with the agility and strength of youth. And immediately he
"took up the bed, and went out in the presence of all, so that all were
amazed and glorified God, saying, 'We never saw anything like this!'"
Mark 2:12.

It required nothing less than creative power to restore health to that
decaying body. The same voice that spoke life to man created from the
dust of the earth had spoken life to the dying paralytic. And the same power
that gave life to the body had renewed his heart. He who at creation "spoke,
and it was," who "commanded, and it stood fast" (Psalm 33:9), had spoken
life to the soul dead in trespasses and sins. The healing of the body was an
evidence of the power that had renewed the heart. Christ commanded the
paralytic to arise and walk, "'that you may know,'" He said, "'that the Son
of Man has power on earth to forgive sins.'"

Healing for Soul and Body

The paralytic found in Christ healing for both soul and body. He needed
health of soul before he could appreciate health of body. Before the physical malady could be healed, Christ must bring relief to the mind and cleanse
the soul from sin. This lesson should not be overlooked. Thousands today
who are suffering from physical disease are, like the paralytic, longing for
the message, "Your sins are forgiven." The burden of sin, with its unrest
and unsatisfied desires, is the foundation of their maladies. They can find
no relief until they come to the Healer of the soul. The peace that He alone
can impart would restore vigor to the mind and health to the body.

The effect produced upon the people by the healing of the paralytic
was as if heaven had opened and revealed the glories of the better world.
As the man who had been cured passed through the throng, blessing God
at every step and bearing his burden as if it were a feather's weight, the
people stepped back to give him room. With awe-stricken faces they gazed
upon him, whispering softly among themselves, "'We have seen strange
things today!'" Luke 5:26.

In the home of the paralytic there was great rejoicing when he returned
to his family, carrying with ease the couch upon which he had been borne
slowly from their presence only a short time before. They gathered around
with tears of joy, hardly daring to believe their eyes. He stood before them
in the full vigor of manhood. Those arms that they had seen lifeless were
quick to obey his will. The flesh that had been pallid and shrunken was
now fresh and ruddy. He walked with a firm, free step. Joy and hope were
written in every feature of his face, and an expression of purity and peace
had taken the place of the marks of sin and suffering.

Glad thanksgiving went up from that home, and God was glorified through His Son, who had restored hope to the hopeless and strength to the stricken one. This man and his family were ready to lay down their lives for Jesus. No doubt dimmed their faith, no unbelief marred their allegiance to Him who had brought light into their darkened home.

"Bless the Lord, O my soul;
And all that is within me, bless His holy name!
Bless the Lord, O my soul,
And forget not all His benefits:
Who forgives all your iniquities,
Who heals all your diseases."

Psalm 103:1-3.

Jesus Heals a Paralytic

"Now there is in Jerusalem by the Sheep Gate a pool, which is called in Hebrew, Bethesda, having five porches. In these lay a great multitude of sick people, blind, lame, paralyzed, waiting for the moving of the water." John 5:2, 3.

At certain seasons the water of this pool was agitated, and it was commonly believed that this was the result of supernatural power. It also was believed that after the water was agitated the first person who stepped into the pool would be healed of whatever disease he or she might have. Hundreds of sufferers visited the place, but so great was the crowd when the water was agitated that they rushed forward, trampling underfoot men, women, and children weaker than themselves. Many could not get near the pool. Others, who had succeeded in reaching it, died on its bank. Shelters had been erected about the place to protect the sick from the heat in the day and the cold at night. Some spent the night in these porches, creeping to the edge of the pool day after day, in the vain hope of relief.

Jesus was at Jerusalem. Walking alone, apparently in meditation and prayer, He came to the pool. He saw the wretched sufferers watching for that which they supposed to be their only chance of cure. He longed to exercise His healing power and make every sufferer whole. But it was the Sabbath day. Multitudes were going to the temple for worship, and He knew that such an act of healing would excite the prejudice of the Jews and cut short His work.

But the Savior saw one case of supreme wretchedness—a man who had been a helpless cripple for thirty-eight years. His disease, in a great degree the result of his own evil habits, was looked upon as a judgment from God. Alone and friendless, feeling shut out from God's mercy, the sufferer had passed long years of misery. At the time when it was expected that the water would be agitated, those who pitied his helplessness would carry him to the porches. But at the favored moment he had no one to help him in. He had seen the rippling of the water but had never been able to get farther than the edge of the pool. Others stronger than he would plunge in before him. The poor, helpless sufferer was unable to contend successfully with the scrambling, selfish crowd. His persistent efforts toward the one goal, and his anxiety and continual disappointment, were fast wearing away the little strength he had left.

The sick man was lying on his mat and occasionally lifting his head to gaze at the pool, when a tender, compassionate face bent over him, and the words, "'Do you want to be made well?'" arrested his attention. Hope came to his heart. He felt that in some way he was to receive help. But the glow of encouragement soon faded. He remembered how often he had tried in vain to reach the pool. Now he had little prospect of living till the water would be agitated again. He turned away wearily, saying, "'Sir, I have no man to put me into the pool when the water is stirred up; but while I am coming, another steps down before me.'"

Jesus commands him, "'Rise, take up your bed and walk.'" Verses 6-8. With new hope the sick man looks at Jesus. The expression of His countenance, the tones of His voice, are like no other. Love and power seem to breathe from His very presence. The cripple's faith takes hold upon Christ's word. Without question he sets his will to obey, and as he does, his whole body responds.

Every nerve and muscle thrills with new life, and healthful action comes to his crippled limbs. Springing to his feet, he goes on his way with firm, free step, praising God and rejoicing in his newfound strength.

Jesus had given the palsied man no assurance of divine help. The man might have said, "Lord, if You will make me whole, I will obey Your word." He might have stopped to doubt, and thus have lost his one chance for healing. But no, he believed Christ's word, believed that he was made whole. Immediately he made the effort, and God gave him the power. He willed to walk, and he did walk. Acting on the word of Christ, he was made whole.

By sin we have been separated from the life of God. Our souls are palsied. Of ourselves we are no more capable of living a holy life than was the crippled man capable of walking. Many realize their helplessness. Longing for that spiritual life that will bring them into harmony with God, they are striving to obtain it. But in vain. In despair they cry, "O wretched man that I am! Who will deliver me from this body of death?" Romans 7:24. Let these desponding, struggling ones look up. The Savior is bending over the purchase of His blood, saying with inexpressible tenderness and pity, "Do you want to be made well?" He bids you arise in health and peace.

Do not wait to feel that you are made whole. Believe the Savior's word. Put your will on the side of Christ. Will to serve Him, and in acting upon

His word you will receive strength. Whatever may be the evil practice, the master passion that through long indulgence binds both soul and body, Christ is able and longs to deliver. He will impart life to the soul that is "dead in trespasses." Ephesians 2:1. He will set free the captive that is held by weakness and misfortune and the chains of sin.

The sense of sin has poisoned the springs of life. But Christ says, "I will take your sins; I will give you peace. I have bought you with My blood. You are Mine. My grace shall strengthen your weakened will; your remorse for sin I will remove."

When temptations assail you, when care and perplexity surround you, when, depressed and discouraged, you are ready to yield to despair, look to Jesus, and the darkness that encompasses you will be dispelled by the bright shining of His presence. When sin struggles for the mastery in your soul and burdens the conscience, look to the Savior. His grace is sufficient to subdue sin. Let your grateful heart, trembling with uncertainty, turn to Him. Lay hold on the hope set before you. Christ waits to adopt you into His family. His strength will help your weakness. He will lead you step by step. Place your hand in His, and let Him guide you.

Never feel that Christ is far away. He is always near. His loving presence surrounds you. Seek Him as One who desires you to find Him. He desires you not only to touch His garments but to walk with Him in constant communion.

A Woman Caught in Adultery

The Feast of Tabernacles had just ended. The priests and rabbis at Jerusalem had been defeated in their plottings against Jesus, and, as evening fell, "everyone went to his own house. But Jesus went to the Mount of Olives." John 7:53; 8:1.

From the excitement and confusion of the city, from the eager crowds and the treacherous rabbis, Jesus turned away to the quiet of the olive groves, where He could be alone with God. But in the early morning He returned to the temple, and as the people gathered about Him He sat down and taught them.

Soon He was interrupted. A group of Pharisees and scribes approached Him, dragging with them a terror-stricken woman. With hard, eager voices they accused her of violating the seventh commandment. Pushing her into the presence of Jesus, they said, with a hypocritical display of respect, "'Teacher, this woman was caught in adultery, in the very act. Now Moses, in the law, commanded us that such should be stoned. But what do You say?'" Verses 4, 5.

Their pretended reverence veiled a deep-laid plot to ruin Jesus. If He acquitted the woman, He might be charged with despising the law of Moses.

If He declared her worthy of death, He could be accused to the Romans as one who assumed authority belonging only to them.

Jesus looked upon the scene—the trembling victim in her shame, the hard-faced dignitaries, devoid of pity. His spirit of stainless purity shrank from the spectacle. Giving no sign that He had heard the question, He stooped and, fixing His eyes upon the ground, began to write in the dust.

Impatient at His delay and apparent indifference, the accusers drew nearer, urging Him to give the matter His attention. But as their eyes, following those of Jesus, focused on the pavement at His feet, their voices were silenced. There, traced before them, were the guilty secrets of their own lives.

Rising, and fixing His eyes upon the plotting elders, Jesus said, "'He who is without sin among *you,* let him throw a stone at her first.'" See verse 7. And, stooping down, He continued writing.

He had not set aside the Mosaic law nor infringed upon the authority of Rome. The accusers were defeated. Now, their robes of pretended holiness torn from them, they stood, guilty and condemned, in the presence of infinite purity. Trembling lest the hidden iniquity of their lives should be laid open to the multitude, with bowed heads and downcast eyes they stole away, leaving their victim with the pitying Savior.

Jesus arose and, looking at the woman, said, "'Where are those accusers of yours? Has no one condemned you?' She said, 'No one, Lord.' And Jesus said to her, 'Neither do I condemn you; go and sin no more.'" Verses 10, 11.

The woman had stood before Jesus, cowering with fear. His words, "'He who is without sin among you, let him throw a stone at her first,'" had come to her as a death sentence. She dared not lift her eyes to the Savior's face, but silently awaited her doom. In astonishment she saw her accusers depart speechless and confounded; then those words of hope fell upon her ear, "'Neither do I condemn you; go and sin no more.'" Her heart was melted, and, bowing at the feet of Jesus, she sobbed out her grateful love, and with bitter tears confessed her sins.

This was to her the beginning of a new life, a life of purity and peace, devoted to God. In the uplifting of this fallen soul, Jesus performed a greater miracle than in healing the most grievous physical disease; He cured the spiritual malady that leads to eternal death. This penitent woman became one of His most steadfast followers. With self-sacrificing love and devotion she showed her gratitude for His forgiving mercy. The world had only contempt and scorn for this erring woman, but the Sinless One pitied her weakness and reached to her a helping hand. While the hypocritical Pharisees condemned, Jesus urged her, "'Go and sin no more.'"

Jesus knows the circumstances of every soul. The greater the sinner's guilt, the more he or she needs the Savior. His heart of divine love and sympathy is drawn out most of all for the one who is most hopelessly entangled in the snares of the enemy. With His own blood He has signed the emancipation papers of the race.

Jesus is not willing for those who have been purchased at such a cost to be buffeted about by the enemy. He does not want us to be overcome by temptation and perish. He who curbed the lions in their den and walked with His faithful witnesses amid the fiery flames is just as ready to work in our behalf to subdue every evil in our nature. Today He is standing at the altar of mercy, presenting before God the prayers of those who desire His help. He turns no weeping, contrite soul away. Freely He will pardon all who come to Him for forgiveness and restoration. He bids every trembling soul take courage. Whoever will, may take hold of God's strength and make peace with Him, and He will make peace.

All who turn to Him for refuge, Jesus lifts above the accusing and the strife of tongues. No human being or evil angel can impeach these souls. Christ unites them to His own divine-human nature. They stand beside the great Sin Bearer in the light proceeding from the throne of God.

The blood of Jesus Christ cleanses "from all sin." 1 John 1:7.

"Who shall bring a charge against God's elect? It is God who justifies. Who is he who condemns? It is Christ who died, and furthermore is also risen, who is even at the right hand of God, who also makes intercession for us." Romans 8:33, 34.

Christ showed that He had absolute control over the winds and waves, and over men possessed of demons. He who stilled the tempest and calmed the troubled sea spoke peace to minds distracted and dominated by Satan.

A Demon Rebuked

In the synagogue at Capernaum, while Jesus was speaking of His mission to set free the slaves of sin, He was interrupted by a shriek of terror. A madman rushed forward from among the people, crying out, "'Let us alone! What have we to do with You, Jesus of Nazareth? Did you come to destroy us? I know who You are—the Holy One of God!'" Mark 1:24.

Jesus rebuked the demon, saying, "'Be quiet, and come out of him!' And when the demon had thrown him in their midst, it came out of him and did not hurt him." Luke 4:35.

The cause of this man's affliction was in his own life. He had been fascinated with the pleasures of sin and had thought to make life a grand carnival. Intemperance and frivolity perverted the noble attributes of his nature, and Satan took entire control of him. Remorse came too late. When he would have sacrificed wealth and pleasure to regain control of his life, he had become helpless in the grasp of the evil one.

In the Savior's presence he was roused to long for freedom, but the demon resisted the power of Christ. When the man tried to appeal to Jesus for help, the evil spirit put words into his mouth, and he cried out in an agony of fear. The demoniac partially comprehended that he was in the presence of One who could set him free, but when he tried to come within reach of that mighty hand, another's will held him, another's words were spoken through him.

The conflict between the power of Satan and his own desire for freedom was terrible. It seemed that the tortured man must die in the struggle with the foe that had been the ruin of his life. But the Savior spoke with authority and set the captive free. The man who had been demon possessed stood before the wondering people in the freedom of self-possession.

With glad voice he praised God for deliverance. The eye that had so lately glared with the fire of insanity now beamed with intelligence and overflowed with grateful tears. The people were dumb with amazement. As soon as they recovered speech they exclaimed one to another, "'What is this? What new doctrine is this? For with authority He commands even the unclean spirits, and they obey Him.'" Mark 1:27

Multitudes today are as truly under the power of evil spirits as was the demoniac of Capernaum. All who willfully depart from God's commandments are placing themselves under the control of Satan. Many tamper with evil, thinking that they can break away whenever they please, but they are lured on and on until they find themselves controlled by a will stronger than their own. They cannot escape its mysterious power. Secret sin or master passion may hold them captive as helpless as was the demoniac of Capernaum.

Yet their condition is not hopeless. God does not control our minds without our consent, but all are free to choose what power they want to rule over them. None have fallen so low, none are so vile, but that they may find deliverance in Christ. The demoniac, in place of prayer, could utter only the words of Satan, yet the heart's unspoken appeal was heard. No cry from a soul in need, though it fail of utterance in words, will be unheeded. Those who consent to enter into covenant with God are not left to the power of Satan or to the infirmity of their own nature.

"Shall the prey be taken from the mighty, or the captives of the righteous be delivered? . . . Thus says the Lord: 'Even the captives of the mighty shall be taken away, and the prey of the terrible be delivered; for I will contend with him who contends with you, and I will save your children.'" Isaiah 49:24, 25.

Marvelous will be the transformation made in anyone who by faith opens the door of the heart to the Savior.

Christ Gives Power

Like the twelve apostles, the seventy disciples whom Christ later sent forth received supernatural endowments as a seal of their mission. When their work was completed, they returned with joy, saying, "'Lord, even the demons are subject to us in Your name.'" Jesus answered, "'I saw Satan fall like lightning from heaven.'" Luke 10:17, 18.

Henceforth Christ's followers are to consider Satan as a conquered foe. Upon the cross, Jesus was to gain the victory for them. That victory He desired them to accept as their own. "'Behold,'" He said, "'I give you the authority to trample on serpents and scorpions, and over all the power of the enemy, and nothing shall by any means hurt you.'" Verse 19.

The omnipotent power of the Holy Spirit is the defense of every soul who surrenders to Jesus. Christ will not permit to pass under the enemy's power anyone who in penitence and faith has claimed His protection. It is true that Satan is a powerful being, but, thank God, we have a mighty Savior who expelled the evil one from heaven. Satan is pleased when we magnify his power. Why not talk of Jesus? Why not magnify His power and His love?

The rainbow of promise encircling the throne in heaven is an everlasting testimony that "God so loved the world that He gave His only begotten Son, that whoever believes in Him should not perish but have everlasting life." John 3:16. It testifies to the universe that God will never forsake His children in the struggle with evil. It is an assurance to us of strength and protection as long as the throne itself endures.

Chapter 6

Saved
to Serve

It is morning on the Sea of Galilee. The light of the rising sun touches sea and land as with a benediction of peace. Jesus and His disciples have spent a tempestuous night on the water, but as they step upon the beach they are greeted with a sight more terrible than the storm-tossed sea. From some hiding place among the tombs two madmen rush upon them as if to tear them in pieces. Hanging about these men are parts of chains that they have broken in escaping from confinement. Their flesh is torn and bleeding. Their eyes glare out from their long, matted hair. The very likeness of humanity seems to have been blotted out. They look more like wild beasts than like men.

The disciples and their companions run away in terror, but presently they notice that Jesus is not with them, and they turn to look for Him. He is standing where they left Him. He who stilled the tempest, who has met Satan before and conquered him, does not flee before demons. When the men, gnashing their teeth and foaming at the mouth, approach Him, Jesus raises that hand which has beckoned the waves to rest, and the men can come no nearer. They stand before Him, raging but helpless.

With authority He commands the unclean spirits to come out of them. The unfortunate men realize that here is One who can save them from the tormenting demons. They fall at the Savior's feet to ask for His mercy. But when their lips open, the demons speak through them, crying, "'What have we to do with You, Jesus, You Son of God? Have You come here to torment us?'" Matthew 8:29.

The evil spirits are forced to release their victims, and a wonderful change comes over the demoniacs. Light shines into their minds. Their eyes beam with intelligence. Their countenances, long deformed into the image of Satan, become suddenly mild. The bloodstained hands are quiet. The men lift their voices in praise to God.

Meanwhile the demons, cast out from their human habitations, have entered into a herd of swine and driven them to destruction by drowning. The keepers of the swine hurry away to spread the news, and the whole population flock to meet Jesus. The two demoniacs have been the terror of the country. Now they are clothed and in their right mind, sitting at the feet of Jesus, listening to His words and glorifying the name of Him who has made them whole. But those who witness this wonderful scene do not rejoice. The loss of the swine seems to them of greater importance than the deliverance of these captives of Satan. In terror they throng about Jesus, pleading with Him to leave. And He complies, taking ship at once for the opposite shore.

Far different is the feeling of the restored demoniacs. They want to be with their Deliverer. In His presence they feel secure from the demons that have tormented their lives and wasted their manhood. As Jesus is about to enter the boat, they keep close to His side, kneel at His feet, and beg Him to remain near them so they may listen to His words. But Jesus bids them go home and tell what great things the Lord has done for them.

Here is a work for them to do—to go to a heathen home and tell of the blessings they have received from Jesus. It is hard for them to be separated from the Savior. Great difficulties will face them as they associate with their heathen countrymen. And their long isolation from society seems to have disqualified them for this work. But as soon as Jesus points out their duty, they are ready to obey.

Not only did they tell their own households and neighbors about Jesus, they went throughout Decapolis, everywhere declaring His power to save and describing how He had freed them from the demons.

Though the people of Gergesa had not received Jesus, He did not abandon them to the darkness they had chosen. When they asked Him to leave, they had not heard His words. They did not know what they were rejecting. Therefore He sent the light to them by those to whom they would not refuse to listen.

In causing the destruction of the swine, it was Satan's purpose to turn the people away from the Savior and prevent the preaching of the gospel in that region. But this very occurrence roused the country as nothing else could have done, and directed attention to Christ. Though the Savior Himself departed, the men whom He had healed remained as witnesses to His power. Those who had been mediums of the prince of darkness became channels of light, messengers of the Son of God. When Jesus later returned to Decapolis, the people flocked about Him, and for three days thousands from all the surrounding country heard the message of salvation.

The two restored demoniacs were the first missionaries whom Christ sent to teach the gospel in the region of Decapolis. These men had listened to His words for a short time only. Not one sermon from His lips had fallen upon their ears. They could not instruct the people as the disciples who had been with Christ daily were able to do. But they could tell what they knew— what they themselves had seen, and heard, and felt of the Savior's power. This is what everyone can do whose heart has been touched by the grace of God. This is the witness for which our Lord calls, and for want of which the world is perishing.

The gospel is to be presented not as a lifeless theory but as a living force to change the life. God would have His servants bear testimony to the fact that through His grace all may possess Christlikeness of character and rejoice in the assurance of His great love. He would have us bear testimony to the fact that He cannot be satisfied until all who will accept salvation are reclaimed and reinstated in their holy privileges as His sons and daughters.

He freely accepts even those whose course has been most offensive to Him. When they repent, He imparts to them His divine Spirit and sends them forth into the camp of the disloyal to proclaim His mercy. Souls who have been degraded into instruments of Satan are still, through the power of Christ, transformed into messengers of righteousness and are sent forth to tell how great things the Lord has done for them and has had compassion on them.

Personal Experience and Witness Are Important

After the woman of Capernaum had been healed by the touch of faith, Jesus desired her to acknowledge the blessing she had received. The gifts that the gospel offers are not to be secured by stealth or enjoyed in secret.

> "'You are My witnesses,' says the Lord,
> 'That I am God.'"
> Isaiah 43:12.

Our confession of His faithfulness is Heaven's chosen agency for revealing Christ to the world. We are to acknowledge His grace as made known through His people of old, but that which will be most effectual is the testimony of our own experience. We are witnesses for God as we reveal in ourselves the working of a power that is divine. Every individual has a life distinct from all others and an experience differing essentially from theirs. God desires that our praise shall ascend to Him, marked with our own individuality. These precious acknowledgments to the praise of the glory of His grace, when supported by a Christlike life, have an irresistible power that works for the salvation of souls.

It is for our own benefit to keep every gift of God fresh in our memory. By this means our faith is strengthened to claim and receive more blessings. There is greater encouragement for us in the least blessing we ourselves receive from God than in all the accounts we can read of the faith and experience of others. Souls that respond to the grace of God shall be like a watered garden. Their health shall spring forth speedily; their light shall rise in obscurity, and the glory of the Lord shall be seen upon them.

"What shall I render to the Lord
For all His benefits toward me?"

"Who can utter the mighty acts of the Lord?
Or can declare all His praise?"

"Oh, give thanks to the Lord!
Call upon His name;
Make known His deeds among the peoples.
Sing to Him, sing psalms to Him;
Talk of all His wondrous works."
     Psalm 116:12; 106:2; 105:1, 2. (See also Psalm 45:17;
     56:11-13; 63:3-7; 71:5, 6, 22-24; 104:33, 34.)

Those Who Receive Are to Give

The gospel invitation is not to be narrowed down and presented to only a select few who, we suppose, will do us honor if they accept it. The message is to be given to all. When God blesses His children, it is not for their sake alone, but for the world's sake. As He bestows His gifts on us, it is that we may multiply them by imparting.

No sooner had the Samaritan woman at Jacob's well found the Savior than she brought others to Him. She proved herself a more effective missionary than His own disciples. The disciples saw nothing in Samaria to indicate that it was an encouraging field. Their thoughts were fixed upon a great work to be done in the future. They did not see that right around them was a harvest to be gathered. But through the woman whom they despised a whole cityful were brought to hear Jesus. She carried the light at once to her countrymen.

This woman represents the working of a practical faith in Christ. Every true disciple is born into the kingdom of God as a missionary. No sooner does a person come to know the Savior than he or she desires to make others acquainted with Him. The saving and sanctifying truth cannot be shut up in the heart. Anyone who drinks of the living water becomes a fountain of life.

The receiver becomes a giver. The grace of Christ in the soul is like a spring in the desert, welling up to refresh all. It makes those who are ready to perish eager to drink of the water of life. In doing this we receive a greater blessing than if we work merely to benefit ourselves. It is in working to spread the good news of salvation that we are brought near to the Savior.

Of those who receive His grace the Lord says: " 'I will make them and the places all around My hill a blessing; and I will cause showers to come down in their season; there shall be showers of blessing.' " Ezekiel 34:26.

"On the last day, that great day of the feast, Jesus stood and cried out, saying, 'If anyone thirsts, let him come to Me and drink. He who believes in Me, as the Scripture has said, out of his heart will flow rivers of living water.' " John 7:37, 38.

Those who receive are to impart to others. From every direction are coming calls for help. God calls upon men and women to minister gladly to others. Immortal crowns are to be won. The kingdom of heaven is to be gained. The world, perishing in ignorance, is to be enlightened.

" 'Do you not say, "There are still four months, and then comes the harvest"? Behold, I say to you, lift up your eyes and look at the fields, for they are already white for harvest! And he who reaps receives wages, and gathers fruit for eternal life.' " John 4:35, 36.

For three years the disciples had before them the wonderful example of Jesus. Day by day they walked and talked with Him, hearing His words of cheer to the weary and heavy-laden, and seeing the manifestations of His power in behalf of the sick and afflicted. When the time came for Him to leave, He gave them grace and power to carry forward His work in His name. They were to shed abroad the light of His gospel of love and healing. And the Savior promised that His presence would be with them always. Through the Holy Spirit He would be even nearer than when He walked visibly among them.

The work that the disciples did, we also are to do. Every follower of Christ is to be a missionary. In sympathy and compassion we are to minister to those in need of help, with unselfish earnestness trying to lighten the woes of suffering humanity.

All may find something to do. None need feel that there is no place where they can work for Christ. The Savior identifies Himself with every child of humanity. That we might become members of the heavenly family, He became a member of the earthly family. He is the Son of man, and thus a brother to every son and daughter of Adam. His followers are not to feel themselves detached from the perishing world around them. They are a part of the great web of humanity, and heaven looks upon them as brothers and sisters to sinners as well as to saints.

Millions upon millions of human beings, in sickness and ignorance and sin, have never so much as heard of Christ's love for them. If our condition and theirs were to be reversed, what would we want them to do for us? All this, so far as lies in our power, we are to do for them. Christ's rule of life by which every one of us must stand or fall in the judgment is, "'Whatever you want men to do to you, do also to them.'" Matthew 7:12.

By all that has given us advantage over another—be it education and refinement, nobility of character, Christian training, or religious experience—we are in debt to those less favored, and so far as lies in our power we are to minister to them. If we are strong, we are to hold up the hands of the weak.

Angels of glory who live in the presence of the Father in heaven delight to minister to His little ones. Angels are ever present where they are most needed—with those who have the hardest battles with self to fight, and whose surroundings are the most discouraging. Weak and trembling souls who have many objectionable traits of character are their special charge. That which selfish hearts would regard as humiliating service—to minister to those who are wretched and in every way inferior in character—is the work of the pure, sinless beings from the courts above.

Walking and Working With Jesus

Jesus did not consider heaven a place to be desired while we were lost. He left the heavenly courts for a life of reproach and insult and a death of shame. He who was rich in heaven's priceless treasure became poor, that through His poverty we might be rich. We are to follow in the path that He walked.

Everyone who becomes a child of God should henceforth look upon himself or herself as a link in the chain let down to save the world, one with Christ in His plan of mercy, going forth with Him to seek and save the lost.

Many feel that it would be a great privilege to visit the scenes of Christ's life on earth, to walk where He walked, to look upon the lake and its shorelines where He loved to teach, and the hills and valleys on which His eyes so often rested. But we need not go to Nazareth, to Capernaum, or to Bethany to walk in the steps of Jesus. We shall find His footprints beside the sickbed, in the homes of the poor, in the crowded streets of the great cities, and in every place where there are human hearts in need of consolation.

We are to feed the hungry, clothe the naked, and comfort the suffering and afflicted. We are to minister to the despairing and inspire hope in the hopeless.

The love of Christ, manifested in unselfish ministry, will be more effective in reforming criminals than will the night stick or the court of justice. These are necessary to strike terror to the lawbreaker, but loving missionaries can do more than this. Often the heart that hardens under reproof will melt under the love of Christ.

Missionaries can not only relieve physical illnesses, they can lead sinners to the Great Physician, who can cleanse the soul from the leprosy of sin. Through His servants, God designs that the sick, the unfortunate, and those possessed of evil spirits shall hear His voice. Through His human agencies He desires to be a comforter such as the world knows not.

The Savior has given His precious life in order to establish a church capable of ministering to the suffering, the sorrowful, and the tempted. A company of believers may be poor, uneducated, and unknown, yet in Christ they may do a work in the home, in the community, and even in "the regions beyond," whose results shall be as far-reaching as eternity.

To Christ's followers today, no less than to the first disciples, these words are spoken: "'All authority has been given to Me in heaven and on earth. Go therefore, and make disciples of all the nations.'" "'Go into all the world and preach the gospel to every creature.'" Matthew 28:18, 19; Mark 16:15.

And for us also is the promise of His presence, "'Lo, I am with you always, even to the end of the age.'" Matthew 28:20.

Today no curious multitudes flock to the desert to see and hear Christ. His voice is not heard in the busy streets. No cry sounds from the wayside, "Jesus of Nazareth is passing by." Luke 18:37. Yet this word is true today. Christ walks unseen through our streets. He comes to our homes with messages of mercy. He waits to cooperate with all who are seeking to minister in His name. He is in the midst of us, to heal and to bless, if we will receive Him.

"How beautiful upon the mountains
Are the feet of him who brings good news,
Who proclaims peace,
Who brings glad tidings of good things,
Who proclaims salvation,
Who says to Zion, 'Your God reigns! . . .'
Break forth into joy, sing together,
You waste places. . . .
For the Lord has comforted His people. . . .
The Lord has made bare His holy arm
In the eyes of all the nations;
And all the ends of the earth shall see
The salvation of our God."

Isaiah 52:7, 9, 10. (See also Isaiah 49:8, 9.)

The Work of the Physician

C *h a p t e r 7*

The Co-working
of the Divine
and the Human

In the ministry of healing, physicians are to be co-workers with Christ. The Savior ministered to both soul and body. The gospel that He taught was a message of spiritual life and of physical restoration. Deliverance from sin and the healing of disease were linked together. The same ministry is committed to Christian physicians. They are to unite with Christ in relieving both the physical and spiritual needs of humanity. They are to be messengers of mercy to the sick, bringing to them a remedy for the diseased body and the sin-sick soul.

Christ is the true head of the medical profession. The chief Physician, He is at the side of every God-fearing practitioner who works to relieve human suffering. While physicians use nature's remedies for physical disease, they should point patients to Him who can relieve the maladies of both soul and body. That which physicians can only aid in doing, Christ accomplishes. They endeavor to assist nature's work of healing; Christ Himself is the healer. Physicians seek to preserve life; Christ imparts life.

The Source of Healing

The Savior in His miracles revealed the power that is continually at work in behalf of human beings, to sustain and to heal them. Through the agencies of nature God is working, day by day, hour by hour, moment by moment, to keep us alive, to build up and restore us. When any part of the body sustains injury, a healing process is begun at once; nature's agencies are set at work to restore soundness. But the power working through these agencies is the power of God. All life-giving power is from Him. When people recover from disease, it is God who restores them.

Sickness, suffering, and death are the work of an antagonistic power. Satan is the destroyer; God is the restorer.

The words spoken to Israel are true today of those who recover health of body or health of soul. "'I am the Lord who heals you.'" Exodus 15:26.

The desire of God for every human being is expressed in the words, "Beloved, I pray that you may prosper in all things and be in health, just as your soul prospers." 3 John 2.

It is God who "forgives all your iniquities, who heals all your diseases, who redeems your life from destruction, who crowns you with lovingkindness and tender mercies." Psalm 103:3, 4.

When Christ healed disease, He warned many of the afflicted ones, "'Sin no more, lest a worse thing come upon you.'" John 5:14. Thus He taught that they had brought disease upon themselves by transgressing the laws of God, and that health could be preserved only by obedience.

Physicians should teach their patients to cooperate with God in the work of restoration. Disease is the result of sin. The laws of nature, as truly as the precepts of the Decalogue, are divine, and only in obedience to them can health be preserved or recovered. Many who are suffering as the result of hurtful practices might be restored to health if they would do what they could for their own restoration. They need to be taught that every practice that destroys the physical, mental, or spiritual energies is sin, and that health is to be secured through obedience to the laws that God has established for the good of all humanity.

A physician who sees a patient suffering from disease caused by improper eating and drinking or other wrong habits, yet neglects to tell him or her of this, is doing injury to a fellow being. Drunkards, maniacs, those who are given over to licentiousness, all should be told clearly and distinctly that suffering results from sin. Those who understand the principles of life should be in earnest in striving to counteract the causes of disease. Seeing the continual conflict with pain, working constantly to alleviate suffering, how can physicians hold their peace? Are they benevolent and merciful if they do not teach strict temperance as a remedy for disease?

Let it be made plain that the way of God's commandments is the way of life. God has established the laws of nature, but His laws are not arbitrary exactions. Every "You shall not," whether in physical or in moral law, implies a promise. If we obey it, blessings will follow. God never forces us to do right, but He endeavors to save us from the evil and lead us to the good.

Consider the laws that were taught to the Israelites. God gave His people definite instruction in regard to their habits of life. He made known to them the laws relating to both physical and spiritual well-being, and on condition of obedience He assured them, "'The Lord will take away from you all sickness.'" "'Set your hearts on all the words which I testify among you today.'" "For they are life to those who find them, and health to all their flesh." Deuteronomy 7:15; 32:46; Proverbs 4:22.

God desires us to reach the standard of perfection made possible for us by the gift of Christ. He calls upon us to make our choice on the right side, to connect with heavenly agencies, to adopt principles that will restore in us the divine image. In His written Word and in the great book of nature He has revealed the principles of life. It is our work to obtain a knowledge of these principles, and by obedience to cooperate with Him in restoring health to the body as well as to the soul.

People need to learn that the blessings of obedience, in their fullness, can be theirs only as they receive the grace of Christ. It is His grace that gives us power to obey the laws of God. It is this that enables us to break the bondage of evil habit. This is the only power that can make us and keep us steadfast in the right path.

When the gospel is received in its purity and power, it is a cure for the disorders that originated in sin. The Sun of Righteousness arises "with healing in His wings." Malachi 4:2. Not all that this world bestows can heal a broken heart, or impart peace of mind, or remove care, or banish disease. Fame, genius, talent—all are powerless to cheer the sorrowful heart or restore the wasted life. The life of God in the soul is our only hope.

The love that Christ diffuses through the whole being is a life-giving power. Every vital part—the brain, the heart, the nerves—it touches with healing. By it the highest energies of the being are roused to activity. It frees the soul from the guilt and sorrow, the anxiety and care, that crush the life forces. With it come serenity and composure. In the soul it implants joy that nothing earthly can destroy—joy in the Holy Spirit—health-giving, life-giving joy.

Our Savior's words, "'Come to Me, . . . and I will give you rest'" (Matthew 11:28), are a prescription for the healing of physical, mental, and spiritual ills. Though people have brought suffering on themselves by their own wrongdoing, He regards them with pity. In Him they may find help. He will do great things for those who trust in Him.

Although for ages sin has been strengthening its hold on the human race, although through falsehood and trickery Satan has cast the black shadow of his interpretation upon the Word of God and has caused people to doubt His goodness, yet the Father's mercy and love have not ceased to flow earthward in rich currents. If human beings would open the windows of the soul heavenward in appreciation for the divine gifts, a flood of healing virtue would pour in.

Seek Constantly to Improve

Physicians who desire to be acceptable co-workers with Christ will strive to become efficient in every feature of their work. They will study diligently, that they may be well qualified for the responsibilities of their profession, and will constantly endeavor to reach a higher standard, seeking for increased knowledge, greater skill, and deeper discernment. Every physician should realize that he or she who does weak, inefficient work is not only doing injury to the sick but also doing injustice to other physicians. The physician who is satisfied with a low standard of skill and knowledge not only belittles the medical profession, but does dishonor to Christ, the Chief Physician.

Those who find that they are unfitted for medical work should choose some other employment. Those who are well adapted to care for the sick but whose education and medical qualifications are limited would do well to minister faithfully as nurses. By patient service under skillful physicians they may be constantly learning, and by improving every opportunity to acquire knowledge they may in time become fully qualified for the work of a physician. Let the younger physicians, "as workers together with him [the Chief Physician], . . . receive not the grace of God in vain, . . . giving no offense in any thing, that the ministry [of the sick] be not blamed: but in all things approving ourselves as the ministers of God." 2 Corinthians 6:1-4, KJV.

God's purpose for us is that we shall ever move upward. The true medical missionary physician will be an increasingly skillful practitioner. Talented Christian physicians, having superior professional ability, should be encouraged to engage in the service of God in places where they can educate and train others to become medical missionaries.

Physicians should gather to their souls the light of the Word of God. They should make continual growth in grace. With them, religion is not to be merely one influence among others, it is to be an influence dominating all others. They are to act from high, holy motives—motives that are powerful because they proceed from the One who gave His life to furnish us with power to overcome evil. If physicians faithfully and diligently strive to make themselves efficient in their profession, if they consecrate themselves to the service of Christ and take time to search their own hearts, they will understand how to grasp the mysteries of their sacred calling. They may so discipline and educate themselves that all within the sphere of their influence will see the excellence of the education and wisdom gained by a person who is connected with the God of wisdom and power.

In no place is a closer fellowship with Christ needed than in the work of the physician. Anyone who would rightly perform the physician's duties must daily and hourly live a Christian life. The life of the patient is in the hands of the physician. One careless diagnosis, one wrong prescription, in a critical case, or one unskillful movement of the hand during surgery, and a life may be sacrificed, a soul's probation ended. How solemn the thought! How important that the physician shall be ever under the control of the divine Physician!

The Savior is willing to help all who call upon Him for wisdom and clearness of thought. And who needs wisdom and clearness of thought more than does the physician, upon whose decisions so much depends? Let the one who is trying to prolong life look in faith to Christ to direct his or her every movement. The Savior will give the necessary tact and skill in dealing with difficult cases.

Seeking God's Help Through Prayer

Wonderful are the opportunities given to the guardians of the sick. In all that is done for the restoration of the sick, let them understand that the physician is seeking to help them cooperate with God in combating disease. Lead them to feel that at every step taken in harmony with the laws of God, they may expect the aid of divine power.

The sick and suffering will have much more confidence in the physician who they are confident loves and fears God. They rely upon his or her words. They feel a sense of safety in the presence and administration of that physician.

Knowing the Lord Jesus, it is the privilege of the Christian health professional to invite His presence into the sickroom by prayer. Before performing critical operations, physicians should ask for the aid of the Great Physician. They should assure the suffering ones that God can bring them safely through the ordeal, that in all times of distress He is a sure refuge for those who trust in Him. The physician who cannot do this loses case after case that otherwise might have been saved. If he or she could speak words that would inspire faith in the sympathizing Savior, who feels every throb of anguish, and could present the needs of the soul to Him in prayer, the crisis would more often be passed safely.

Only He who reads the heart can know with what trembling and terror many patients consent to an operation under the surgeon's hand. They realize their peril. While they may have confidence in the physician's skill, they know it is not infallible. But as they see the physician pray, asking help from God, they are inspired with confidence. Gratitude and trust open the heart to the healing power of God, the energies of the whole being are vitalized, and the life forces triumph.

To the physician as well as to the patient, the Savior's presence is an element of strength. Often the responsibilities and possibilities of the physician's work bring dread upon the spirit. The feverishness of uncertainty and fear would make the hand unskillful. But the assurance that the divine Counselor is present to guide and to sustain imparts quietness and courage. The touch of Christ upon the physician's hand brings vitality, restfulness, confidence, and power.

When the crisis is passed and success is apparent, let a few moments be spent with the patient in prayer. Give expression to your thankfulness for the life that has been spared. As words of gratitude flow from the patient to the physician, let the praise and thanksgiving be directed to God. Tell the patient his life has been spared because he was under the heavenly Physician's protection.

Physicians who follow such a course are leading their patients to the One upon whom they are dependent for life, the One who can save to the uttermost all who come to Him.

Into the medical missionary work should be brought a deep yearning for souls. To the physician equally with the gospel minister is committed the highest trust ever committed to humans. Whether he or she realizes it, every physician is entrusted with the cure of souls.

In their work of dealing with disease and death, physicians too often lose sight of the solemn realities of the future life. In their earnest effort to avert the peril of the body, they forget the peril of the soul. The ones to whom they are ministering may be losing their hold on life. Life's last opportunities are slipping away. These souls the physician must meet again at the judgment seat of Christ.

Often we miss the most precious blessings by neglecting to speak a word in season. If the golden opportunity is not watched for, it will be lost. At the bedside of the sick no word of creed or controversy should be spoken. Let the sufferer be pointed to the One who is willing to save all who come to Him in faith. Earnestly, tenderly strive to help the soul that is hovering between life and death.

Physicians who know that Christ is their personal Savior, because they themselves have been led to the Refuge, know how to deal with the trembling, guilty, sin-sick souls who turn to them for help. They can respond to the inquiry, "What must I do to be saved?" They can tell the story of the Redeemer's love. They can speak from experience of the power of repentance and faith. In simple, earnest words they can present the soul's need to God in prayer and can encourage the sick one also to ask for and accept the mercy of the compassionate Savior. As they thus minister at the bedside of the sick, trying to speak words that will bring help and comfort, the Lord works with them and through them. As the mind of the sufferer is directed to the Savior, peace fills the heart, and the spiritual health that comes is used as the helping hand of God in restoring health to the body.

In attending the sick, the physician will often find opportunity for ministering to friends of the afflicted one. As they watch by the bed of suffering, feeling powerless to prevent the pangs of anguish, their hearts are softened. Often grief concealed from others is expressed to the physician.

Then is the opportunity to point these sorrowing ones to Him who has invited the weary and heavy-laden to come to Him. Often prayer can be offered for and with them, presenting their needs to the Healer of all woes, the Soother of all sorrows.

God's Promises

Physicians have precious opportunities for directing patients to the promises of God's Word. They are to bring from the treasure house things new and old, speaking here and there words of comfort and instruction. Physicians should make their minds a storehouse of fresh thoughts. Let them study the Word of God diligently, that they may be familiar with its promises. Let them learn to repeat the comforting words that Christ spoke during His earthly ministry when giving His lessons and healing the sick. They should talk of Christ's works of healing, of His tenderness and love. Never should they neglect to direct the minds of their patients to Christ, the Chief Physician.

The same power that Christ exercised when He walked visibly on earth is in His Word. It was by His word that Jesus healed disease and cast out demons. By His word He stilled the sea and raised the dead, and the people bore witness that His word was with power. He spoke the word of God, as He had spoken to all the prophets and teachers of the Old Testament. The whole Bible is a manifestation of Christ.

The Scriptures are to be received as God's word to us, not written merely but spoken. When the afflicted ones came to Christ, He saw not only those who asked for help but all who throughout the ages should come to Him in like need and with like faith. When He said to the paralytic, "'Son, be of good cheer; your sins are forgiven you,'" and when He said to the woman of Capernaum, "'Daughter, be of good cheer; your faith has made you well. Go in peace,'" He spoke to other afflicted, sin-burdened ones who should seek His help. Matthew 9:2; Luke 8:48.

So with all the promises of God's Word. In them He is speaking to us individually, speaking as directly as if we could hear His voice. It is in these promises that Christ communicates to us His grace and power. They are leaves from that tree which is "for the healing of the nations." Revelation 22:2. Received, assimilated, they are to be the strength of the character, the inspiration and sustenance of the life. Nothing else can have such healing power. Nothing else can impart the courage and faith that give vital energy to the whole being.

To one who stands trembling with fear on the brink of the grave, to the soul weary of the burden of suffering and sin, let the physician, as opportunity presents itself, repeat the words of the Savior—for all the words of Holy Writ are His: "'Fear not, for I have redeemed you; I have called you by your name; you are Mine. When you pass through the waters, I will be with you; and through the rivers, they shall not overflow you. When you walk through the fire, you shall not be burned, nor shall the flame scorch you. For I am the Lord your God, the Holy One of Israel, your Savior. . . . Since you were precious in My sight, you have been honored, and I have loved you.'" "'I, even I, am He who blots out your transgressions for My own sake; and I will not remember your sins.'" "'Fear not, for I am with you.'" Isaiah 43:1-4, 25, 5.

"As a father pities his children, so the Lord pities those who fear Him. For He knows our frame; He remembers that we are dust." Psalm 103:13, 14.

"If we confess our sins, He is faithful and just to forgive us our sins and to cleanse us from all unrighteousness." 1 John 1:9.

"'I have blotted out, like a thick cloud, your transgressions, and like a cloud, your sins. Return to Me, for I have redeemed you.'" Isaiah 44:22.

"'I have loved you with an everlasting love; therefore with lovingkindness I have drawn you.'" Jeremiah 31:3.

"'Let not your heart be troubled.'" "'Peace I leave with you, My peace I give to you; not as the world gives do I give to you. Let not your heart be troubled, neither let it be afraid.'" John 14:1, 27.

"'Look to Me, and be saved, all you ends of the earth!'" Isaiah 45:22.

"'He Himself took our infirmities and bore our sicknesses.'" "He was wounded for our transgressions, He was bruised for our iniquities; the chastisement for our peace was upon Him, and by His stripes we are healed." Matthew 8:17; Isaiah 53:5.

C h a p t e r   8

The Physician
an Educator

True physicians are educators. They recognize their responsibility not only to the sick who are under their direct care but also to the communities in which they live. They stand as guardians of both physical and moral health. It is their endeavor not only to teach right methods for the treatment of the sick but to encourage right habits of living and to spread a knowledge of right principles.

Education in health principles was never more needed than now. Notwithstanding wonderful progress in many lines relating to the comforts and conveniences of life, even to sanitary matters and to the treatment of disease, the decline in physical vigor and power of endurance is alarming. It demands the attention of all who have at heart the well-being of the human family.

Our artificial civilization is encouraging evils that are destructive of sound principles. Custom and fashion are at war with nature. The practices they enjoin and the indulgences they foster are steadily lessening both physical and mental strength. They are bringing upon the race an intolerable burden. Intemperance and crime, disease and wretchedness are everywhere.

Avoid Poisonous Drugs

Many transgress the laws of health through ignorance, and they need instruction. But the greater number know better than they do. They need to be impressed with the importance of making their knowledge a guide of life. The physician has many opportunities both of imparting a knowledge of health principles and of showing the importance of putting them in practice. By right instruction he or she can do much to correct evils that are working untold harm.

A practice that is laying the foundation of a vast amount of disease and of even more serious evils is the free use of poisonous drugs. When attacked by disease, many of the sick will not take the trouble to search out the cause of their illness. Their chief aim is to rid themselves of pain and inconvenience. So they resort to patent nostrums, of whose real properties they know little, or they apply to a physician for some remedy to counteract the result of their misdoing, but with no thought of making a change in their unhealthful habits. If immediate benefit is not realized, they try another medicine, and then another. Thus the evil continues.

People need to be taught that drugs do not cure disease. True, they sometimes afford present relief, and the patient appears to recover as the result of their use. This improvement is because nature has sufficient vital force to expel the poison and correct the conditions that caused the disease. Health is recovered in spite of the drug. But in most cases the drug only changes the form and location of the disease. Often the effect of the poison seems to be overcome for a time, but the results remain in the system and work great harm at some later period.

By the use of poisonous drugs many bring upon themselves lifelong illness, and many lives are lost that might be saved by the use of natural methods of healing. The poisons contained in many so-called remedies create habits and appetites that result in ruin to both soul and body. Many of the popular nostrums called patent medicines, and even some of the drugs prescribed by physicians, act a part in laying the foundation of the liquor habit, the opium habit, the morphine habit that are a terrible curse to society.

The only hope of improving things is to educate the people in right principles. Physicians should teach the people that restorative power is not in drugs but in nature. In case of sickness, the cause should be ascertained. Unhealthful conditions should be changed, wrong habits corrected. Then nature is to be assisted in her effort to expel impurities and to reestablish right conditions in the system.

Natural Remedies

Pure air, sunlight, abstemiousness, rest, exercise, proper diet, the use of water, trust in divine power—these are the true remedies. Every person should have a knowledge of nature's remedial agencies and how to apply them. It is essential both to understand the principles involved in the treatment of the sick and to have a practical training that will enable one to apply this knowledge.

The use of natural remedies requires an amount of care and effort that many are not willing to give. Nature's process of healing and upbuilding is gradual, and to impatient people it seems slow. The surrender of hurtful indulgences requires sacrifice, but in the end it will be found that nature, unrestricted, does her work wisely and well. Those who persevere in obedience to her laws will be rewarded with health of body and health of mind.

Too little attention is generally given to preserving one's health. It is far better to prevent disease than to know how to treat it when contracted. It is the duty of every person, for his or her own sake, and for the sake of humanity, to be informed in regard to the laws of life and to obey them conscientiously. All need to become acquainted with that most wonderful of all organisms, the human body. They should understand the functions of the various organs and the dependence of one upon another for the healthy action of all. They should study the influence of the mind on the body and of the body on the mind, and the laws by which they are governed.

Training for Life's Conflict

We cannot be reminded too often that health does not depend on chance. It is a result of obedience to law. This is recognized by competitors in athletic games and contests requiring strength. These men and women make the most careful preparation. They submit to thorough training and strict discipline. Every physical habit is carefully regulated. They know that neglect, excess, or carelessness, which weakens or cripples any organ or function of the body, would guarantee defeat.

How much more important is such carefulness to ensure success in the conflict of life. It is not make-believe battles in which we are engaged. We are waging a warfare upon which hang eternal results. We have unseen enemies to meet. Evil angels are trying to dominate every human being. Whatever injures one's health not only lessens physical vigor but tends to weaken the mental and moral powers. Indulgence in any unhealthful practice makes it more difficult for a person to discriminate between right and wrong, and hence more difficult to resist evil. It increases the danger of failure and defeat.

"Those who run in a race all run, but one receives the prize." 1 Corinthians 9:24. In the warfare in which we are engaged, all may win who will discipline themselves by obedience to right principles. The practice of these principles in the details of life is often looked upon as unimportant—a matter too trivial to demand attention. But in view of the issues at stake, nothing with which we have to do is small. Every act casts its weight into the scale that determines life's victory or defeat. The Scripture urges us, "Run in such a way that you may obtain." Verse 24.

With our first parents, intemperate desire resulted in the loss of Eden. Temperance in all things has more to do with our restoration to Eden than people realize.

Pointing to the self-denial practiced by the contestants in the ancient Greek games, the apostle Paul writes: "Everyone who competes for the prize is temperate in all things. Now they do it to obtain a perishable crown, but we for an imperishable crown. Therefore I run thus: not with uncertainty. Thus I fight: not as one who beats the air. But I discipline my body and bring it into subjection, lest, when I have preached to others, I myself should become disqualified." Verses 25-27.

The progress of reform depends on a clear recognition of fundamental truth. Danger lurks in a narrow philosophy and a hard, cold orthodoxy, but on the other hand, there is great danger in a careless liberalism. The foundation of all enduring reform is the law of God. We are to present in clear, distinct lines the need of obeying this law. Its principles must be kept before the people. They are as everlasting and inexorable as God Himself.

One of the most deplorable effects of the original apostasy was that human beings lost the power of self-control. Only as this power is regained can there be real progress.

The body is the only medium through which the mind and the soul are developed for the upbuilding of character. For this reason the adversary of souls directs his temptations to enfeebling and degrading the physical powers. His success here means the surrender to evil of the whole being. The tendencies of our physical nature, unless under the dominion of a higher power, are sure to work ruin and death.

The body is to be brought into subjection. The higher powers of the being are to rule. The passions are to be controlled by the will, which is itself to be under the control of God. The kingly power of reason, sanctified by divine grace, is to bear sway in our lives.

The requirements of God must be brought home to the conscience. Men and women must be awakened to the duty of self-mastery, the need of purity, freedom from every depraving appetite and defiling habit. They need to be impressed with the fact that all their powers of mind and body are gifts from God, and are to be preserved in the best possible condition for His service.

In ancient Israel's sacrificial ritual, which was the gospel in symbol, no blemished offering could be brought to God's altar. The sacrifice that was to represent Christ must be spotless. The Word of God points to this as an illustration of what His children are to be—"a living sacrifice," "holy and without blemish," "acceptable to God." Romans 12:1; Ephesians 5:27.

Apart from divine power, no genuine reform can be effected. Human barriers against natural and cultivated tendencies are but as a sandbank against the torrent. Not until the life of Christ becomes a vitalizing power in our lives can we resist the temptations that assail us from within and from without.

Christ came to this world and lived the law of God that we might have perfect mastery over the natural inclinations that corrupt the soul. The Physician of soul and body, He gives victory over warring lusts. He has provided every facility, so that human beings may possess completeness of character.

When one surrenders to Christ, the mind is brought under the control of the law—the royal law—that proclaims liberty to every captive. By becoming one with Christ, we are made free. Subjection to the will of Christ means restoration to perfect manhood and womanhood.

Obedience to God is liberty from the slavery of sin, deliverance from human passion and impulse. Human beings may stand as conquerors, conquerors of their own inclinations, conquerors of principalities and powers, and of "the rulers of the darkness of this age," and of "spiritual hosts of wickedness in the heavenly places." Ephesians 6:12.

Nowhere is such instruction as this more needed than in the home, and nowhere will it be productive of greater good. Parents are involved with the very foundation of habit and character. The reformatory movement must begin in presenting to them the fact that the principles of the law of God bear upon both physical and moral health. Show that obedience to God's Word is our only safeguard against the evils that are sweeping the world to destruction. Make plain the responsibility of parents not only for themselves but for their children. They are giving to their children an example either of obedience or of transgression. By their example and teaching, the destiny of their households is decided. The children will be what their parents make them.

If parents could trace the result of their actions and could see how, by their example and teaching, they perpetuate and increase the power of sin or the power of righteousness, they certainly would make a change. Many would turn away from tradition and custom, and accept the divine principles of life.

Power of Example

The physician who ministers in the homes of the people, watching at the bedside of the sick, relieving their distress, bringing them back from the borders of the grave, speaking hope to the dying, wins a place in their confidence and affection such as is granted to few others. Not even to the minister of the gospel are committed possibilities so great or an influence so far-reaching.

The physician's example, no less than his or her teaching, should be a positive power on the right side. The cause of reform calls for men and women whose life practice is an illustration of self-control. It is our practice of the principles we inculcate that gives them weight. The world needs a practical demonstration of what the grace of God can do in restoring to human beings their lost sovereignty, giving them mastery of themselves. There is nothing that the world needs so much as a knowledge of the gospel's saving power revealed in Christlike lives.

Physicians are continually brought into contact with those who need the strength and encouragement of a right example. Many people are weak in moral power. They lack self-control and are easily overcome by temptation. Physicians can help these souls only as they reveal in their own lives a strength of principle that enables them to triumph over every injurious habit and defiling lust. Their lives must reveal the working of a power that is divine. If they fail here, however forcible or persuasive their words may be, their influence will tell for evil.

Multitudes seek medical advice and treatment who have become moral wrecks through their own wrong habits. They are bruised and weak and wounded, feeling their folly and their inability to overcome. Such ones should have nothing in their surroundings to encourage a continuance of the thoughts and feelings that have made them what they are. They need to breathe an atmosphere of purity, of high and noble thought. How terrible the responsibility when those who should give them a right example are themselves enthralled by hurtful habits, their influence giving added strength to temptation!

Physicians and the Temperance Work

Many come under physicians' care who are ruining soul and body by the use of tobacco or intoxicating drink. Physicians who are true to their responsibility must point out to these patients the cause of their suffering. But if they themselves are users of tobacco or intoxicants, what weight will be given to their words? With the consciousness of their own indulgence in mind, will they not hesitate to point out the plague spot in the life of their patients? While using these things themselves, how can they convince the youth of their injurious effects?

How can physicians stand in the community as examples of purity and self-control, how can they be effectual workers in the temperance cause, while they themselves are indulging a vile habit? How can they minister acceptably at the bedside of the sick and the dying when their very breath is offensive, smelling of liquor or tobacco?

With disordered nerves and a brain clouded by the use of narcotic poisons, how can one be true to the trust placed in him or her as a skillful physician? How impossible for such a one to comprehend quickly or act swiftly with precision!

If physicians do not observe the laws that govern their own being, if they choose selfish gratification above soundness of mind and body, do they not thereby declare themselves unfit to be entrusted with the responsibility of human lives?

However skilled and faithful physicians may be, there is in their experience much of apparent discouragement and defeat. Often their work fails of accomplishing that which they long to see accomplished. Though health is restored to their patients, it may be no real benefit to them or to the world. Many recover health, only to repeat the indulgences that invited disease. With the same eagerness as before, they plunge again into the round of self-indulgence and irrational conduct. The physician's work for them seems like effort thrown away.

Christ had the same experience, yet He did not cease His efforts for even one suffering soul. Of the ten lepers who were cleansed, only one appreciated the gift, and he was a stranger and a Samaritan. For the sake of that one, Christ healed the ten. If physicians meet with no better success than that of the Savior, let them learn a lesson from the Chief Physician. Of Christ it is written, "He will not fail nor be discouraged." "He shall see the travail of His soul, and be satisfied." Isaiah 42:4; 53:11.

If but one soul would have accepted the gospel of His grace, Christ would, to save that one, have chosen His life of toil and humiliation and His death of shame. If through our efforts even one human being is uplifted and ennobled, fitted to shine in the courts of the Lord, should we not rejoice?

Physicians have duties that are arduous and trying. In order to perform them most successfully they need to have a strong constitution and vigorous health. A man or woman who is feeble or diseased cannot endure the exhausting work accompanying to the physician's calling. One who lacks perfect self-control cannot become qualified to deal with all classes of disease.

Often deprived of sleep, neglecting even to eat, cut off in great degree from social enjoyment and religious privileges, the life of physicians seems to lie under a continual shadow. The affliction they see, the dependent mortals longing for help, their contact with the depraved, make the heart sick and well-nigh destroy confidence in humanity. In the battle with disease and death, every energy is taxed to the limit of endurance. The reaction from this terrible strain tests the character to the utmost. Then it is that temptation has greatest power. More than those in any other calling, physicians are in need of self-control, purity of spirit, and that faith which takes hold on heaven. For the sake of others and for their own sake, they cannot afford to disregard physical law. Recklessness in physical habits tends to recklessness in morals.

The physician's only safety is, under all circumstances, to act from principle, strengthened and ennobled by a firmness of purpose found only in God. Both men and women are to stand in the moral excellence of His character. Day by day, hour by hour, moment by moment, they are to live as in the sight of the unseen world. As did Moses, they must endure "as seeing Him who is invisible."

Righteousness has its root in godliness. No one can steadily maintain before others a pure, forceful life unless that life is hidden with Christ in God. The greater the interaction with humanity, the closer must be the communion of the heart with heaven. The more urgent the duties and the greater the responsibilities, the greater the physician's need of divine power. Time must be redeemed from things temporal for meditation upon things eternal. He or she must resist an encroaching world, which would so press upon the soul as to separate one from the Source of strength. Above all other people, physicians should, by prayer and study of the Scriptures, place themselves under the protecting shield of God. They are to live in hourly contact and conscious communion with the principles of truth, righteousness, and mercy that reveal God's attributes within the soul.

Just to the degree in which the Word of God is received and obeyed will it impress with its potency and touch with its life every spring of action, every phase of character. It will purify every thought, regulate every desire. Those who make God's Word their trust will be courageous and strong. They will rise above all baser things into an atmosphere free from defilement.

When a person is in fellowship with God, the unswerving purpose that preserved Joseph and Daniel amidst the corruption of heathen courts will make the life one of unsullied purity. The robe of character will be spotless. In his or her life the light of Christ will be undimmed. Above such a person the bright and morning Star will appear shining steadfastly in changeless glory.

Such a life will be an element of strength in the community. It will be a barrier against evil, a safeguard to the tempted, a guiding light to those who, amidst difficulties and discouragements, are seeking the right way.

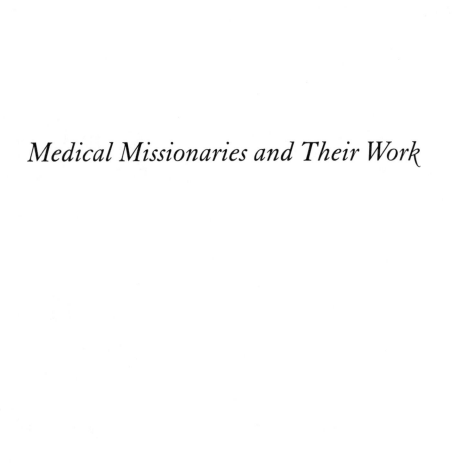

Medical Missionaries and Their Work

Chapter 9

Teaching
and Healing

When Christ sent out the twelve disciples on their first missionary tour, He said to them, "'As you go, preach, saying, "The kingdom of heaven is at hand." Heal the sick, cleanse the lepers, raise the dead, cast out demons. Freely you have received, freely give.'" Matthew 10:7, 8.

To the seventy sent forth later He said: "'Whatever city you enter, . . . heal the sick there, and say to them, "The kingdom of God has come near to you."'" Luke 10:8, 9. The presence and power of Christ was with them, and "the seventy returned with joy, saying, 'Lord, even the demons are subject to us in Your name.'" Verse 17.

After Christ's ascension, the same work was continued. The scenes of His own ministry were repeated. "From the surrounding cities" there came a multitude "to Jerusalem, bringing sick people and those who were tormented by unclean spirits, and they were all healed." Acts 5:16.

The disciples "went out and preached everywhere, the Lord working with them." "Philip went down to the city of Samaria and preached Christ to them. And the multitudes with one accord heeded the things spoken by Philip. . . . For unclean spirits . . . came out of many who were possessed; and many who were paralyzed and lame were healed. And there was great joy in that city." Mark 16:20; Acts 8:5-8.

Work of the Disciples

Luke, the writer of the Gospel that bears his name, was a medical missionary. In the Scriptures he is called "the beloved physician." Colossians

4:14. The apostle Paul heard of his skill as a physician and sought him out as one to whom the Lord had entrusted a special work. He secured his cooperation, and for some time Luke accompanied him in his travels from place to place. After a time, Paul left Luke at Philippi, in Macedonia. Here he continued to work for several years, both as a physician and as a teacher of the gospel. In his service as a physician he ministered to the sick and then prayed for the healing power of God to rest upon the afflicted ones. Thus the way was opened for the gospel message. Luke's success as a physician gained for him many opportunities for preaching Christ among the heathen.

It is the divine plan that we shall work as the disciples worked. Physical healing is bound up with the gospel commission. In the work of the gospel, teaching and healing are never to be separated.

The work of the disciples was to spread a knowledge of the gospel. To them was committed the work of proclaiming to all the world the good news that Christ brought to humankind. That work they accomplished for the people of their time. To every nation under heaven the gospel was carried in a single generation.

Giving the gospel to the world is the work that God has committed to those who have taken His name. The gospel is the only antidote for earth's sin and misery. To make known to everyone the message of the grace of God is the first work of all who know its healing power.

When Christ sent forth the disciples with the gospel message, faith in God and His Word had well-nigh departed from the world. The Jewish people professed to have a knowledge of God, but His Word had been set aside for tradition and human speculation. Selfish ambition, love of ostentation, greed of gain absorbed the people's thoughts. As reverence for God departed, compassion toward one another also departed. Selfishness was the ruling principle, and Satan worked his will in the misery and degradation of the human race.

Satanic agencies took possession of people. The bodies of human beings, made for the dwelling place of God, became the habitation of demons. The senses, the nerves, the organs of humans were worked by supernatural agencies in the indulgence of the vilest lust. The very stamp of demons was impressed upon the countenances of men and women. Human faces reflected the expression of the legions of evil with which the people were possessed.

What is the condition in the world today? Is not faith in the Bible as effectually destroyed by the higher criticism and speculation of today as it was by tradition and rabbinism in the days of Christ? Do not greed, ambition, and love of pleasure have as strong a hold on human hearts now as they had then? In the so-called Christian world, even in the professed churches of Christ, how few are governed by Christian principles. In business, social, domestic, even religious circles, how few make the teachings of Christ the rule of daily living. Is it not true that "justice is turned back, and righteousness stands afar off; . . . equity cannot enter . . . and he who departs from evil makes himself a prey"? Isaiah 59:14, 15.

We are living in the midst of an "epidemic of crime," at which thoughtful, God-fearing people everywhere stand aghast. The corruption that prevails is beyond the power of the human pen to describe. Every day brings fresh revelations of political strife, bribery, and fraud. Every day brings its heart-sickening record of violence and lawlessness, of indifference to human suffering, of brutal, fiendish destruction of human life. Every day testifies to the increase of insanity, murder, and suicide. Who can doubt that satanic agencies are at work with increased activity to distract and corrupt the mind, and to defile and destroy the body?

And while the world is filled with these evils, the gospel is too often presented in so indifferent a manner as to make little impression upon the consciences and lives of people. Everywhere hearts are crying out for something that they do not have. They long for a power that will give them mastery over sin, a power that will deliver them from the bondage of evil, a power that will give health and life and peace. Many who once knew the power of God's Word have been living where there is no recognition of God, and they long for the divine presence.

The world today needs what it needed two thousand years ago—a revelation of Christ. A great work of reform is demanded, and it is only through the grace of Christ that the work of restoration—physical, mental, and spiritual—can be accomplished.

Personal Ministry Needed

Christ's method alone will give true success in reaching the people. The Savior mingled with people as one who desired their good. He showed sympathy for them, ministered to their needs, and won their confidence. Then He invited them, "Follow Me."

We need to come close to the people by personal effort. If we would give less time to sermonizing and more time to personal ministry, greater results would be seen. The poor are to be relieved, the sick cared for, the sorrowing and the bereaved comforted, the ignorant instructed, the inexperienced counseled. We are to weep with those who weep and to rejoice with those who rejoice. Accompanied by the power of persuasion, the power of prayer, the power of the love of God, this work will not, cannot, be without fruit.

We should ever remember that the object of medical missionary work is to point sin-sick men and women to the Man of Calvary, who takes away the sin of the world. By holding Him in view, they will be changed into His likeness. We are to encourage the sick and suffering to look to Jesus and live.

Let the workers keep Christ, the Great Physician, constantly before those to whom disease of body and soul has brought discouragement. Point them to the One who can heal both physical and spiritual disease. Tell them of the One who is touched with the feeling of their infirmities. Encourage them to place themselves in the care of Him who gave His life to make it possible for them to have life eternal. Talk of His love. Tell of His power to save.

This is the high duty and precious privilege of the medical missionary. And personal ministry often prepares the way for this. God often reaches hearts through our efforts to relieve physical suffering.

Medical missionary work is the pioneer work of the gospel. In the ministry of the Word and in the medical missionary work, the gospel is to be preached and practiced.

In almost every community there are large numbers who do not listen to the preaching of God's Word or attend any religious service. But they can be reached by the gospel as missionary nurses bring relief of their physical needs in their homes. As missionary nurses care for the sick and relieve the distress of the poor, they will find many opportunities to pray with them, read from God's Word, and speak to them of the Savior. They can pray with and for those who do not have the strength of will to control the appetites that passion has degraded. They can bring a ray of hope into the lives of the defeated and disheartened. Their unselfish love, manifested in acts of disinterested kindness, will make it easier for these suffering ones to believe in the love of Christ.

Many have no faith in God and have lost confidence in their fellow mortals. But they appreciate acts of sympathy and helpfulness. As they see one with no inducement of earthly praise or compensation come into their homes, ministering to the sick, feeding the hungry, clothing the naked, comforting the sad, and tenderly pointing all to Him of whose love and pity the human worker is but the messenger—as they see this, their hearts are touched. Gratitude springs up. Faith is kindled. They see that God cares for them, and they are prepared to listen as His Word is opened.

Whether in foreign missions or in the home field, all workers, both men and women, will gain much more ready access to the people and will find their usefulness greatly increased if they are able to minister to the sick. When every other door of access is closed, women who go for service in lands afar may thus find opportunity for giving the gospel to the women of these lands. All gospel workers should know how to give simple treatments that do much to relieve pain and remove disease.

Teaching Health Principles

Gospel workers should also be able to give instruction in the principles of healthful living. There is sickness everywhere, and most of it might be prevented by attention to the laws of health. The people need to see the bearing that health principles have on their well-being, both for this life and for the life to come. They need to be awakened to their responsibility for the human habitation designed by their Creator to be His dwelling place, and over which He desires them to be faithful stewards. They need to be impressed with the truth conveyed in the inspired words of Paul:

"You are the temple of the living God. As God has said: 'I will dwell in them, and walk among them. I will be their God, and they shall be My people.'" 2 Corinthians 6:16.

Thousands need and would gladly receive instruction concerning simple methods of treating the sick—methods that take the place of poisonous drugs. There is great need of instruction in regard to reform in diet. Wrong habits of eating and the use of unhealthful food are in no small degree responsible for the intemperance, crime, and wretchedness that curse the world.

In teaching health principles, keep before the mind the great object of reform—that its purpose is to secure the highest development of body, mind, and soul. Show that the laws of nature, being the laws of God, are designed for our good. Obedience to them promotes happiness in this life and aids in preparation for the life to come.

Lead the people to study God's love and wisdom as revealed in the works of nature. Lead them to study that marvelous organism, the human system, and the laws by which it is governed. Those who perceive the evidences of God's love, who understand something of the wisdom and beneficence of His laws, and the results of obedience, will come to regard their duties and obligations from an altogether different point of view. Instead of looking upon obedience to the laws of health as a matter of sacrifice or self-denial, they will regard it as it really is—an inestimable blessing.

Gospel workers should feel that giving instruction in the principles of healthful living is a part of their appointed work. Of this work there is great need, and the world is open for it.

Everywhere there is a tendency to substitute the work of organizations for individual effort. Human wisdom tends to consolidation, to centralization, to the building up of great churches and institutions. Multitudes leave to institutions and organizations the work of benevolence; they excuse themselves from contact with the world, and their hearts grow cold. They become self-absorbed and unimpressible. Love for God and humanity dies out of the soul.

Christ commits to His followers an individual work—a work that cannot be done by proxy. Ministry to the sick and poor, the giving of the gospel to the lost, is not to be left to committees or organized charities. Individual responsibility, individual effort, personal sacrifice, is the requirement of the gospel.

" ' "Go out into the highways and hedges, and compel them to come in," ' " is Christ's command, " ' "that My house may be filled." ' " He brings men and women into touch with those whom they seek to benefit. " 'Bring to your house the poor who are cast out,' " He says. " 'When you see the naked, that you cover him.' " " 'They will lay hands on the sick, and they will recover.' " Luke 14: 23; Isaiah 58:7; Mark 16:18. Through direct contact, through personal ministry, the blessings of the gospel are to be communicated.

In giving light to His people anciently, God did not work through only one class. Daniel was a prince of Judah. Isaiah also was of the royal line. David was a shepherd, Amos a herdsman. Zechariah was a captive from Babylon, Elisha a farmer. The Lord raised up as His representatives prophets and princes, the noble and the lowly, and taught them the truths to be given to the world.

To everyone who becomes a partaker of His grace the Lord appoints a work for others. Individually we are to stand in our lot and place, saying, " 'Here am I! Send me.' " Isaiah 6:8. Upon the minister of the Word, the missionary nurse, the Christian physician, the individual Christian, whether merchant or farmer, professional or mechanic—the responsibility rests upon all. It is our work to reveal to earth's inhabitants the gospel of salvation. Every enterprise in which we engage should be a means to this end.

Those who take up their appointed work will not only be a blessing to others, they themselves will be blessed. The consciousness of duty well done will have a reflex influence upon their own souls. The despondent will forget their despondency, the weak will become strong, the ignorant intelligent, and all will find an unfailing helper in Him who has called them.

The Church a Training School

The church of Christ is organized for service. Its watchword is ministry. Its members are soldiers, to be trained for conflict under the Captain of their salvation. Christian ministers, physicians, and teachers have a broader work than many have recognized. They are not only to minister to the people, they are to teach the people to minister. They should not only give instruction in right principles, they should educate their hearers to impart these principles. Truth that is not lived, that is not imparted, loses its life-giving power, its healing virtue. Its blessing can be retained only as it is shared.

The monotony of our service for God needs to be broken up. Every church member should be engaged in some line of service for the Master. Some cannot do as much as others, but everyone should do his or her utmost to roll back the tide of disease and distress that is sweeping over our world. Many would be willing to work if they were taught how to begin. They need to be instructed and encouraged.

Every church should be a training school for Christian workers. Its members should be taught how to give Bible readings, how to conduct and teach Sabbath school classes, how best to help the poor, care for the sick, and work for the unconverted. There should be schools of health, cooking schools, and classes in various lines of Christian help work. There should be not only teaching but actual work under experienced instructors. The teachers should lead the way in working among the people, and others, uniting with them, will learn from their example. One example is worth more than many precepts.

Let all cultivate their physical and mental powers to the utmost of their ability, that they may work for God where His providence shall call them. The same grace that came from Christ to Paul and Apollos, that distinguished them for spiritual excellencies, will today be imparted to devoted Christian missionaries. God desires His children to have intelligence and knowledge, that with unmistakable clearness and power His glory may be revealed in our world.

Consecrated workers who are educated can do service in a greater variety of ways and can accomplish more extensive work than can those who are uneducated. Their discipline of mind places them on vantage ground. But those who have neither great talents nor extensive education may minister acceptably. God will use anyone who is willing to be used. It is not the most brilliant or most talented person whose work produces the greatest and most lasting results. Men and women are needed who have heard a message from heaven. The most effective workers are those who respond to the invitation, "'Take My yoke upon you and learn from Me.'" Matthew 11:29.

It is heart missionaries that are needed. A person whose heart God touches is filled with a great longing for those who have never known His love. Their condition impresses him or her with a sense of personal woe. Taking life in hand, the heaven-sent, heaven-inspired messenger goes forth to do a work in which angels can cooperate.

If those to whom God has entrusted great talents of intellect put these gifts to a selfish use, they will be left, after a period of trial, to follow their own way. God will take workers who do not appear to be so richly endowed, who have not large self-confidence, and He will make the weak strong, because they trust in Him to do for them that which they cannot do for themselves. God will accept their wholehearted service and will Himself make up their deficiencies.

The Lord has often chosen for His co-workers people who have obtained only a limited formal education. These men and women have applied their powers most diligently, and the Lord has rewarded their industry, their thirst for knowledge, and their fidelity to His work. He has seen their tears and heard their prayers. As His blessing came to the captives in the courts of Babylon, so He gives wisdom and knowledge to His workers today.

Men and women deficient in school education, lowly in social position, have, through the grace of Christ, sometimes been wonderfully successful in winning souls for Him. The secret of their success was their confidence in God. Daily they learned of Him who is wonderful in counsel and mighty in power.

Such workers are to be encouraged. The Lord brings them into connection with those of more marked ability, to fill up the gaps that others leave. Their quickness to see what is to be done, their readiness to help those in need, their kind words and deeds open doors of usefulness that otherwise would remain closed. They come close to those in trouble, and the persuasive influence of their words has power to draw many trembling souls to God. Their work shows what thousands of others might do if they only would.

A Broader Life

Nothing will arouse a self-sacrificing zeal and broaden and strengthen the character as will engaging in work for others. Many professed Christians, in joining a church, think only of themselves. They wish to enjoy church fellowship and pastoral care. They become members of large and prosperous churches and are content to do little for others. In this way they are robbing themselves of the most precious blessings. Many would be greatly benefited by sacrificing their pleasant, comfortable situation. They need to go where their energies will be called out in Christian work and they can learn to bear responsibilities.

Trees that are crowded together do not become healthy and strong. The gardener transplants them that they may have room to develop. A similar work would benefit many of the members of large churches. They need to be placed where their energies will be called forth in active Christian effort. They are losing their spiritual life, becoming dwarfed and inefficient, because they lack self-sacrificing work for others. Transplanted to some missionary field, they would grow strong and vigorous.

But none need wait until called to some distant field before beginning to help others. Doors of service are open everywhere. All around us are those who need our help. The widow, the orphan, the sick and dying, the heartsick, the discouraged, the ignorant, and the outcast are on every hand.

We should feel it our special duty to work for those in our neighborhood. Study how you can best help those who take no interest in religious things. As you visit your friends and neighbors, show an interest in both their spiritual and temporal welfare. Speak to them of Christ as a sin-pardoning Savior. Invite your neighbors to your home, and read with them from the precious Bible and from books that explain its truths. Invite them to unite with you in song and prayer. In these little gatherings, Christ Himself will be present, as He has promised, and hearts will be touched by His grace.

Church members should educate themselves to do this work. This is just as essential as to save the benighted souls in foreign countries. While some feel burdened to win souls in distant lands, the many who are at home should feel the burden of precious souls who are around them, and work diligently for their salvation.

Many regret that they are living a narrow life. They themselves can make their life broad and influential if they will. Those who love Jesus with heart and mind and soul, and their neighbors as themselves, have a wide field in which to use their ability and influence.

None should pass by little opportunities, looking for larger work. You might do successfully the small work but fail utterly in attempting the larger work and become discouraged. It is by doing with your might what you find to do that you will develop aptitude for larger work. It is by slighting the daily opportunities, by neglecting the little things right at hand, that many become fruitless and withered.

Do not depend upon human aid. Look beyond human beings to the One appointed by God to bear our griefs, carry our sorrows, and supply our necessities. Taking God at His word, make a beginning wherever you find work to do, and move forward with unfaltering faith. It is faith in Christ's presence that gives strength and steadfastness. Work with unselfish interest, with painstaking effort, with persevering energy.

In fields where the conditions are so objectionable and disheartening that many are unwilling to go to them, remarkable changes have been made by the efforts of self-sacrificing workers. Patiently and perseveringly they worked, not relying on human power but on God, and His grace sustained them. The amount of good thus accomplished will never be known in this world, but blessed results will be seen in the great hereafter.

Self-Supporting Missionaries

In many places self-supporting missionaries can work successfully. It was as a self-supporting missionary that the apostle Paul spread the knowledge of Christ throughout the world. While daily teaching the gospel in the great cities of Asia and Europe, he worked at the trade of a craftsman to sustain himself and his companions. His parting words to the elders of Ephesus, showing his method of labor, have precious lessons for every gospel worker:

"'You know,'" he said, "'in what manner I always lived among you . . . and how I kept back nothing that was helpful, but proclaimed it to you, and taught you publicly and from house to house. . . . I have coveted no one's silver or gold or apparel. Yes, you yourselves know that these hands have provided for my necessities, and for those who were with me. I have shown you in every way, by laboring like this, that you must support the weak. And remember the words of the Lord Jesus, that He said, "It is more blessed to give than to receive." '" Acts 20:18-35.

Many today, if imbued with the same spirit of self-sacrifice, could do a good work in a similar way. Let two or more start out together in evangelistic work. Let them visit the people, praying, singing, teaching, explaining the Scriptures, and ministering to the sick. Some can sustain themselves as literature evangelists. Others, like the apostle, can work at some handicraft or in other lines of effort. As they move forward in their lives, realizing their helplessness but humbly depending upon God, they gain a blessed experience. The Lord Jesus goes before them, and among the wealthy and the poor they find favor and help.

Those who have been trained for medical missionary work in foreign countries should be encouraged to go without delay and begin work among the people, learning the language as they work. Very soon they will be able to teach the simple truths of God's Word.

Throughout the world, messengers of mercy are needed. There is a call for Christian families to go into communities that are in darkness and error, to go to foreign fields, to become acquainted with the needs of the people, and to work for the cause of the Master. If such families would settle in the dark places of the earth, and let the light of Christ's life shine out through them, what a noble work might be accomplished.

This work requires self-sacrifice. While many are waiting to have every obstacle removed, the work they might do is left undone, and multitudes are dying without hope and without God. Some people, for the sake of commercial advantage or to acquire scientific knowledge, will venture into unsettled regions and cheerfully endure sacrifice and hardship, but how few for the sake of others are willing to move their families into regions that are in need of the gospel.

To reach the people, wherever they are, and whatever their position or condition, and to help them in every way possible—this is true ministry. By such effort you may win hearts and open a door of access to perishing souls.

In all your work remember that you are bound up with Christ, a part of the great plan of redemption. The love of Christ, in a healing, life-giving current, is to flow through your life. As you seek to draw others within the circle of His love, let the purity of your language, the unselfishness of your service, the joyfulness of your demeanor bear witness to the power of His grace. Present so pure and righteous a representation of Him that the world shall see Him in His beauty.

It is of little use to try to reform others by attacking what we may regard as wrong habits. Such effort often results in more harm than good.

In Christ's conversation with the Samaritan woman, instead of disparaging Jacob's well, He presented something better. "'If you knew the gift of God,'" He said, "'and who it is who says to you, "Give Me a drink," you would have asked Him, and He would have given you living water.'" John 4:10. He turned the conversation to the treasure He could give, offering the woman something better than she possessed, even living water, the joy and hope of the gospel.

This is an illustration of the way in which we are to work. We must offer people something better than that which they possess, even the peace of Christ. We must tell them of God's holy law, the transcript of His character and an expression of that which He wishes them to become. Show them how infinitely superior to the fleeting joys and pleasures of the world is the imperishable glory of heaven. Tell them of the freedom and rest to be found in the Savior. "'Whoever drinks of the water that I shall give him will never thirst,'" He declared. Verse 14.

Lift up Jesus, like John, crying, "'Behold! The Lamb of God who takes away the sin of the world!'" John 1:29. He alone can satisfy the craving of the heart and give peace to the soul.

Reformers Should Reflect Christ

Of all people in the world, reformers should be the most unselfish, the most kind, the most courteous. The true goodness of unselfish deeds should be seen in their lives. Workers who manifest a lack of courtesy, who show impatience at the ignorance or waywardness of others, who speak hastily or act thoughtlessly, may close the door to hearts, making it impossible for the gospel to reach them.

As the dew and the soft showers fall upon withering plants, so let words fall gently when seeking to win people from error. God's plan for us is first to reach the heart. We are to speak the truth in love, trusting in Him to give it power for reforming the life. The Holy Spirit will apply to the soul the word that is spoken in love.

By nature we are self-centered and opinionated. But when we learn the lessons that Christ desires to teach us, we become partakers of His nature and live His life. The wonderful example of Christ, the matchless tenderness with which He entered into the feelings of others, weeping with those who wept, rejoicing with those who rejoiced, must have a deep influence upon the character of all who follow Him in sincerity. By kindly words and acts they will try to make the path easy for weary feet.

"'The Lord God has given Me the tongue of the learned, that I should know how to speak a word in season to him who is weary.'" Isaiah 50:4.

All around us are afflicted souls. Here and there, everywhere, we may find them. Let us search out these suffering ones and speak a word in season to comfort their hearts. Let us ever be channels through which shall flow the refreshing waters of compassion.

In all our associations it should be remembered that in the experience of others there are chapters sealed from mortal sight. On the pages of memory are sad histories that are sacredly guarded from curious eyes. There stand registered long, hard battles with trying circumstances, perhaps troubles in the home life, that day by day weaken courage, confidence, and faith. Those who are fighting the battle of life at great odds may be strengthened and encouraged by little attentions that cost only a loving effort. To such, the strong, helpful grasp of the hand by a true friend is worth more than gold or silver. Words of kindness are as welcome as the smile of angels.

Multitudes are struggling with poverty, compelled to work hard for low pay, and able to secure only the barest necessities of life. Toil and deprivation, with no hope of better things, make their burden very heavy. When pain and sickness are added, the load is almost unbearable. Careworn and oppressed, they know not where to turn for relief. Sympathize with them in their trials, their heartaches, and disappointments. This will open the way for you to help them. Speak to them of God's promises, pray with and for them, inspire them with hope.

Words of cheer and encouragement spoken when the soul is sick and the pulse of courage is low—these are regarded by the Savior as if spoken to Himself. As hearts are cheered, the heavenly angels look on in pleased recognition.

From age to age the Lord has been working to awaken in human souls a sense that all belong to God's family, that all are brothers and sisters. Be co-workers with Him. While distrust and alienation are pervading the world, Christ's disciples are to reveal the spirit that reigns in heaven.

Speak as He would speak, act as He would act. Constantly reveal the sweetness of His character. Reveal that wealth of love which underlies all His teachings and all His dealings with mortal beings. The humblest workers, in cooperation with Christ, may touch chords whose vibrations shall ring to the ends of the earth and make melody throughout eternal ages.

Heavenly intelligences are waiting to cooperate with human instrumentalities, that they may reveal to the world what human beings may become, and what, through union with the Divine, may be accomplished for the saving of souls that are ready to perish. There is no limit to the usefulness of one who, putting self aside, makes room for the working of the Holy Spirit upon the heart and lives a life wholly consecrated to God.

All who consecrate body, soul, and spirit to His service will be constantly receiving a new endowment of physical, mental, and spiritual power. The inexhaustible supplies of heaven are at their command. Christ gives them the breath of His own Spirit, the life of His own life. The Holy Spirit puts forth its highest energies to work in mind and heart. Through the grace given us we may achieve victories that, because of our own erroneous and preconceived opinions, our defects of character, our smallness of faith, have seemed impossible.

To all who offer themselves to the Lord for service, withholding nothing, is given power to attain measureless results. For these men and women, God will do great things. He will work upon their minds so that, even in their mortal state, there shall be seen in their lives a fulfillment of the promise of the future state.

"The wilderness and the wasteland shall be glad for them;
And the desert shall rejoice and blossom as the rose;
It shall blossom abundantly and rejoice,
Even with joy and singing. . . .
Then the eyes of the blind shall be opened,
And the ears of the deaf shall be unstopped.
Then the lame shall leap like a deer,
And the tongue of the dumb sing.
For waters shall burst forth in the wilderness,
And streams in the desert.
The parched ground shall become a pool,
And the thirsty land springs of water. . . .
A highway shall be there, and a road,
And it shall be called the Highway of Holiness. . . .
The redeemed shall walk there,
And the ransomed of the Lord shall return,
And come to Zion with singing,
With everlasting joy on their heads.
They shall obtain joy and gladness,
And sorrow and sighing shall flee away."
Isaiah 35:1-10.

Helping
the Tempted

Not because we first loved Him did Christ love us, but "while we were still sinners" He died for us. He does not treat us as we deserve. Although our sins merit condemnation, He does not condemn us. Year after year He has borne with our weakness and ignorance, with our ingratitude and waywardness. Despite our wanderings, our hardness of heart, our neglect of His Holy Word, His hand is stretched out still.

Grace is an attribute of God exercised toward undeserving human beings. We did not seek for it, but it was sent in search of us. God rejoices to extend His grace to us, not because we are worthy but because we are so utterly unworthy. Our only claim to His mercy is our great need.

The Lord God through Jesus Christ holds out His hand all the day long in invitation to the sinful and fallen. He will receive all. He welcomes all. It is His glory to pardon the chief of sinners. He will deliver the captive. He will lower the golden chain of His mercy to the lowest depths of human wretchedness and lift up the debased soul contaminated with sin.

Every human being is the object of loving interest to Him who gave His life that He might bring sinners back to God. Guilty and helpless souls, liable to be destroyed by the arts and snares of Satan, are cared for as a shepherd cares for the sheep of his flock.

The Savior's example is to be the standard of our service for the tempted and the erring. We are to manifest toward others the same interest, tenderness, and longsuffering that He has manifested toward us. "'As I have loved you,'" He says, "'that you also love one another.'" John 13:34. If Christ lives in us, we shall reveal His unselfish love toward all with whom we have to do. As we see men and women in need of sympathy and help, we shall not ask, "Are they worthy?" but, "How can I benefit them?"

Rich and poor, high and low, free and bond are God's heritage. He who gave His life to redeem sinners sees in every human being a value that exceeds finite computation. By the mystery and glory of the cross we are to discern His estimate of the value of the soul. When we do this, we shall feel that human beings, however degraded, have cost too much to be treated with coldness or contempt. We shall realize the importance of working for lost souls, that they may be saved and exalted to the throne of God.

The lost coin in the Savior's parable, though lying in the dirt and rubbish, was still a piece of silver. Its owner wanted to find it because it was of value. So every soul, however degraded by sin, is in God's sight accounted precious. As the coin bore the image and superscription of the reigning power, so human beings at creation bore the image and superscription of God. Though now marred and dim through the influence of sin, the traces of this inscription remain on every soul. God desires to recover that soul and to retrace upon it His own image in righteousness and holiness.

How little do we enter into sympathy with Christ on that which should be the strongest bond of union between us and Him—compassion for depraved, guilty, suffering souls, dead in trespasses and sins! Our inhumanity toward others is our greatest sin. Many think that they are representing the justice of God while they wholly fail to represent His tenderness and His great love. Often the ones whom they treat with sternness and severity are under the stress of temptation. Satan is wrestling with these souls, and harsh, unsympathetic words discourage them and cause them to fall a prey to the tempter's power.

It is a delicate matter to deal with minds. Only He who reads the heart knows how to bring people to repentance. Only His wisdom can give us success in reaching the lost. You may stand up stiffly, feeling, "I am holier than you," and it matters not how correct your reasoning or how true your words; they will never touch hearts. The love of Christ, revealed in word and act, will win its way to the soul when reiterating precepts or arguments would accomplish nothing.

We need more Christlike sympathy not merely for those who appear to us to be faultless but for poor, suffering, struggling souls who are often overtaken in fault, sinning and repenting, tempted and discouraged. We are to go to our fellow mortals, touched, like our merciful High Priest, with the feeling of their infirmities.

It was the outcast, the publican and sinner, the despised of the nations, that Christ called and drew to Himself by His lovingkindness. The one class that He would never countenance was those who stood apart in their self-esteem and looked down on others.

"Go out into the highways and hedges, and compel them to come in," Christ urges us, "that My house may be filled." In obedience to this word we must go to the "heathen" who are near us and to those who are afar off. The "publicans and harlots" must hear the Savior's invitation. Through the kindness and longsuffering of His messengers, the invitation becomes a compelling power to uplift those who are sunken in the lowest depths of sin.

Christian motives demand that we work with a steady purpose, an undying interest, an ever-increasing earnestness for the souls whom Satan is seeking to destroy. Nothing is to chill our earnest, yearning energy for the salvation of the lost.

Mark how all through the Word of God there is manifest the spirit of urgency, of imploring men and women to come to Christ. To draw people to the Savior we must seize every opportunity, in private and in public, presenting every argument, urging every motive of infinite weight. With all our power we must urge them to look to Jesus and to accept His life of self-denial and sacrifice. We must show that we expect them to give joy to the heart of Christ by using every one of His gifts in honoring His name.

Saved by Hope

"We are saved by hope." Romans 8:24, KJV. The fallen must be led to feel that it is not too late for them to repent. Christ honored sinners with His confidence and thus placed them on their honor. Even those who had fallen the lowest He treated with respect. It was a continual pain to Christ to be brought into contact with enmity, depravity, and impurity, but never did He utter one word to show that His sensibilities were shocked or His refined tastes offended. Whatever the evil habits, the strong prejudices, or the overbearing passions of human beings, He met them all with pitying tenderness.

As we partake of His Spirit, we shall regard every person as a brother or sister, with similar temptations and trials, often falling and struggling to rise again, battling with discouragements and difficulties, craving sympathy and help. Then we shall meet them in such a way as not to discourage or repel them, but to awaken hope in their hearts. As they are thus encouraged, they can say with confidence, "Do not rejoice over me, my enemy; when I fall, I will arise; when I sit in darkness, the Lord will be a light unto me." He "pleads my case, and executes justice for me; He will bring me forth to the light, and I will see His righteousness." Micah 7:8, 9.

God "looks on all the inhabitants of the earth;
He fashions their hearts individually."
Psalm 33:14, 15.

He counsels us, in dealing with the tempted and erring, consider "yourself lest you also be tempted." Galatians 6:1. With a sense of our own infirmities, we shall have compassion for the infirmities of others.

"Who makes you differ from another? And what do you have that you did not receive?" "'One is your Teacher, . . . and you are all brethren.'" "Why do you judge your brother? Or why do you show contempt for your brother?" "Therefore let us not judge one another, . . . but rather resolve this, not to put a stumbling block or a cause to fall in our brother's way." 1 Corinthians 4:7; Matthew 23:8; Romans 14:10, 13.

It is always humiliating to have one's errors pointed out. None should make the experience more bitter by needless censure. No one was ever reclaimed by reproach, but many have thus been repelled and have been led to steel their hearts against conviction. A tender spirit, a gentle, winning deportment may save the erring and hide a multitude of sins.

The apostle Paul found it necessary to reprove wrong, but how carefully he tried to show that he was a friend to the erring! How tenderly he explained to them the reason for his action! He made them understand that it cost him pain to give them pain. He showed his confidence and sympathy toward the ones who were struggling to overcome.

"Out of much affliction and anguish of heart," he said, "I wrote to you, with many tears, not that you should be grieved, but that you might know the love which I have so abundantly for you." 2 Corinthians 2:4. "For even if I made you sorry with my letter, I do not regret it; though I did regret it. . . . Now I rejoice, not that you were made sorry, but that your sorrow led to repentance. . . . For observe this very thing, that you sorrowed in a godly manner: What diligence it produced in you, what clearing of yourselves, what indignation, what fear, what vehement desire, what zeal, what vindication! In all things you proved yourselves to be clear in this matter. . . . Therefore we have been comforted." 2 Corinthians 7:8-13.

"I rejoice that I have confidence in you in everything." Verse 16. "I thank my God upon every remembrance of you, always in every prayer of mine making request for you all with joy, for your fellowship in the gospel from the first day until now, being confident of this very thing, that He who has begun a good work in you will complete it until the day of Jesus Christ; just as it is right for me to think this of you all, because I have you in my heart." "Therefore, my beloved and longed-for brethren, my joy and crown, so stand fast in the Lord, beloved." "Now we live, if you stand fast in the Lord." Philippians 1:3-7; 4:1; 1 Thessalonians 3:8.

Paul wrote to these believers as "saints in Christ Jesus," but he was not writing to those who were perfect in character. He wrote to them as men and women who were striving against temptation and who were in danger of falling. He pointed them to "the God of peace who brought up our Lord Jesus from the dead, that great Shepherd of the sheep." He assured them that "through the blood of the everlasting covenant" He will "make you complete in every good work to do His will, working in you what is well pleasing in His sight, through Jesus Christ." Hebrews 13:20, 21.

How to Help the Erring

When people who are at fault become conscious of their error, be careful not to destroy their self-respect. Do not discourage them by indifference or distrust. Do not say, "Before giving them my confidence, I'll wait to see whether they'll hold out." Often this very distrust causes tempted ones to stumble.

We should try to understand the weakness of others. We know little of the heart trials of those who have been bound in chains of darkness and who lack resolution and moral power. Most pitiable is the condition of those who are suffering under remorse. They are as one stunned, staggering, sinking into the dust. They can see nothing clearly. The mind is beclouded, they know not what steps to take. Many a poor soul is misunderstood, unappreciated, full of distress and agony—a lost, straying sheep. The soul cannot find God, yet has an intense longing for pardon and peace.

Utter no word to cause deeper pain! To souls weary of sin but not knowing where to find relief, present the compassionate Savior. Take them by the hand, lift them up, speak to them words of courage and hope. Help them to grasp the hand of the Savior.

We become too easily discouraged over people who do not at once respond to our efforts. Never should we cease to work for a soul while there is one gleam of hope. Precious souls cost our self-sacrificing Redeemer too dear a price to be lightly given up to the tempter's power.

We need to put ourselves in the place of the tempted ones. Consider the power of heredity, the influence of evil associations and surroundings, the power of wrong habits. Can we wonder that under such influences many become degraded? Can we wonder that they should be slow to respond to efforts for their uplifting?

Often, when won to the gospel, those who appeared coarse and unpromising will be among its most loyal adherents and advocates. They are not altogether corrupt. Beneath the rough, forbidding exterior are good impulses that might be reached. Without a helping hand many would never recover themselves, but by patient, persistent effort they may be uplifted. Such need tender words, kind consideration, tangible help. They need the kind of counsel that will not extinguish the faint gleam of courage in the soul. Workers who come in contact with them should consider this.

Some will be found whose minds have been so long debased that they will never in this life become what they might have been under more favorable circumstances. But the bright beams of the Sun of Righteousness may shine into the soul. It is their privilege to have the life that measures with the life of God. Plant in their minds uplifting, ennobling thoughts. Let your life make plain to them the difference between vice and purity, darkness and light. In your example let them read what it means to be a Christian. Christ is able to uplift the most sinful and place them where they will be acknowledged as children of God, joint heirs with Christ to the immortal inheritance.

By the miracle of divine grace, many may be fitted for lives of usefulness. Despised and forsaken, they have become utterly discouraged, and may appear stoical and stolid. But under the ministration of the Holy Spirit, the dull, clouded mind will awake. The slave of sin will be set free. Vice will disappear, and ignorance will be overcome. Through the faith that works by love, the heart will be purified and the mind enlightened.

Working for the Intemperate

Every true reform has its place in the work of the gospel and tends to uplift the soul to a new and nobler life. Especially does temperance reform demand the support of Christian workers. They should call attention to this work and make it a living issue. Everywhere they should present the principles of true temperance and call for people to sign the temperance pledge. Earnest effort should be made in behalf of those who are in bondage to evil habits.

Everywhere there is a work to be done for those who through intemperance have fallen. In the midst of churches, religious institutions, and professedly Christian homes, many of the youth are choosing the path to destruction. Through intemperate habits they bring upon themselves disease, and through greed to obtain money for sinful indulgence they fall into dishonest practices. Health and character are ruined. Aliens from God, outcasts from society, these poor youth feel that they are without hope either for this life or for the life to come. The hearts of the parents are broken. Some people speak of these erring ones as hopeless, but God does not regard them this way. He understands all the circumstances that have made them what they are, and He looks upon them with pity. This is a class that demands help. Never give them occasion to say, "No one cares for my soul."

Among the victims of intemperance are people of all classes and all professions. Men and women of high station, of eminent talents, of great attainments, have yielded to the indulgence of appetite until they are helpless to resist temptation. Some of them who once were rich are without home and friends, in suffering, misery, disease, and degradation. They have lost self-control. Unless a helping hand is held out to them, they will sink lower and lower. With these, self-indulgence is not only a moral sin but a physical disease.

Often in helping the intemperate we must give first attention, as Christ often did, to their physical condition. They need wholesome, unstimulating food and drink, clean clothing, opportunity to secure physical cleanliness. They need to be surrounded with an atmosphere of helpful, uplifting Christian influence. In every city a place should be provided where the slaves of evil habits may receive help to break the chains that bind them. Alcohol is regarded by many as the only solace in trouble, but this need not be if professed Christians, instead of acting the part of the priest and Levite, would follow the example of the good Samaritan.

In dealing with victims of intemperance we must remember that we are not dealing with sane people but with those who for the time being are under the power of a demon. Be patient and forbearing. Think not of the repulsive, forbidding appearance, but of the precious life that Christ died to redeem. As the slave of alcohol awakens to a sense of his degradation, do all in your power to show that you are his friend. Speak no word of censure. Let no act or look express reproach or aversion. Very likely the poor soul curses himself. Help him to rise. Speak words that will encourage faith. Seek to strengthen every good trait in his character. Teach him how to reach upward. Show him that it is possible for him to live in a way that will win the respect of others. Help him to see the value of the talents that God has given him but that he has neglected to improve.

Although the will has been depraved and weakened, there is hope for him. Christ will awaken in the heart higher impulses and holier desires. Encourage him to lay hold of the hope set before him in the gospel. Open the Bible before the tempted, struggling one, and again and again read to him the promises of God. These promises will be to him as the leaves of the tree of life. Patiently continue your efforts until with grateful joy the trembling hand grasps the hope of redemption through Christ.

Do Not Give Up

You must hold fast to those whom you are trying to help, or victory will never be yours. They will be continually tempted to evil. Again and again they will be almost overcome by the craving for strong drink. Again and again they may fall. But do not, because of this, cease your efforts.

They have decided to make an effort to live for Christ, but their will power is weakened, hence they must be carefully guarded by those who watch for souls as they that must give an account. They have lost their self-respect and nobility as human beings, and this they must win back. Many have to battle against strong hereditary tendencies to evil. Unnatural cravings, sensual impulses, were their inheritance from birth. These must be carefully guarded against. Within and without, good and evil are striving for the mastery. Those who have never passed through such experiences cannot know the almost overmastering power of appetite or the fierceness of the conflict between habits of self-indulgence and the determination to be temperate in all things. Over and over the battle must be fought.

Many who are drawn to Christ will not have moral courage to continue the warfare against appetite and passion. But the worker must not be discouraged by this. Is it only those rescued from the lowest depths that backslide?

Remember that you do not work alone. Ministering angels unite in service with every truehearted son and daughter of God. And Christ is the Restorer. The Great Physician Himself stands beside His faithful workers, saying to the repentant soul, "Your sins are forgiven you." Mark 2:5.

Many are the outcasts who will grasp the hope set before them in the gospel and will enter the kingdom of heaven, while others who were blessed with great opportunities and great light that they did not improve will be left in outer darkness.

The victims of evil habits must be aroused to the necessity of making an effort for themselves. Others may put forth the most earnest endeavor to uplift them, the grace of God may be freely offered, Christ may entreat, His angels may minister, but all will be in vain unless they themselves are roused to fight the battle in their own behalf.

The last words of David to Solomon, then a young man, and soon to receive the crown of Israel, were, "'Be strong, . . . and prove yourself a man.'" 1 Kings 2:2. To every child of humanity—candidate for an immortal crown—are these words of inspiration spoken, "Be strong, . . . and prove yourself a man."

The self-indulgent must be led to see and feel that great moral renovation is necessary if they would become Christlike. God calls upon them to arouse and in the strength of Christ win back the God-given nobility that has been sacrificed through sinful indulgence.

Feeling the terrible power of temptation, the drawing of desire that leads to indulgence, many people cry in despair, "I cannot resist evil." Tell them that they can, that they must, resist. They may have been overcome again and again, but it need not be always thus. They are weak in moral power, controlled by the habits of a life of sin. Their promises and resolutions are like ropes of sand. The knowledge of their broken promises and forfeited pledges weakens their confidence in their own sincerity and causes them to feel that God cannot accept them or work with their efforts. But they need not despair.

Those who put their trust in Christ are not to be enslaved by any hereditary or cultivated habit or tendency. Instead of being held in bondage to the lower nature, they are to rule every appetite and passion. God has not left us to battle against evil with only finite strength. Whatever may be our inherited or cultivated tendencies to wrong, we can overcome through the power that He is ready to impart.

The Power of the Will

The tempted one needs to understand the true force of the will. This is the governing power in human beings—the power of decision, of choice. Everything depends on the right action of the will. Desires for goodness and purity are right, so far as they go, but if we stop here they avail nothing. Many will go down to ruin while hoping and desiring to overcome their evil inclinations. They do not yield the will to God. They do not *choose* to serve Him.

God has given us the power of choice; it is ours to exercise. We cannot change our hearts, we cannot control our thoughts, our impulses, our affections. We cannot make ourselves pure, fit for God's service. But we can *choose* to serve God; we can give Him our will. Then He will work in us to will and to do according to His good pleasure. Thus our whole nature will be brought under the control of Christ.

Through the right exercise of the will, an entire change may be made in the life. By yielding the will to Christ, we ally ourselves with divine power. We receive strength from above to hold us steadfast. A pure and noble life, a life of victory over appetite and lust, is possible to all who will unite their weak, wavering human will to the omnipotent, unwavering will of God.

Those who are struggling against the power of appetite should be instructed in the principles of healthful living. They should be shown that violation of the laws of health, by creating diseased conditions and unnatural cravings, lays the foundation of the liquor habit. Only by living in obedience to the principles of health can they hope to be freed from the craving for unnatural stimulants. While they depend upon divine strength to break the bonds of appetite, they are to cooperate with God by obedience to His laws, both moral and physical.

Those who are endeavoring to reform should be provided with employment. None who are able to work should be taught to expect food and clothing and shelter free of cost. For their own sake, as well as for the sake of others, some way should be devised whereby they may return an equivalent for what they receive. Encourage every effort toward self-support. This will strengthen self-respect and a noble independence. And employing mind and body in useful work is essential as a safeguard against temptation.

Disappointments and Dangers

Those who work for the fallen will be disappointed in many who give promise of reform. Many will make but a superficial change in their habits and practices. They are moved by impulse, and for a time may seem to have reformed, but there is no real change of heart. They cherish the same self-love, have the same hungering for foolish pleasures, the same desire for self-indulgence. They have not a knowledge of the work of character building, and they cannot be relied upon as men and women of principle. They have debased their mental and spiritual powers by the gratification of appetite and passion, and this makes them weak. They are fickle and changeable. Their impulses tend toward sensuality. These persons are often a source of danger to others. Being looked upon as reformed men and women, they are trusted with responsibilities and are placed where their influence corrupts the innocent.

Even those who are sincerely seeking to reform are not beyond the danger of falling. They need to be treated with great wisdom as well as tenderness. The disposition to flatter and exalt those who have been rescued from the lowest depths sometimes proves their ruin. The practice of inviting men and women to relate in public the experience of their life of sin is full of danger to both speaker and hearers. To think about and describe scenes of evil corrupts mind and soul. And the prominence given to the rescued ones is harmful to them. Many are led to feel that their sinful life has given them a certain distinction. A love of public acclaim and a spirit of self-trust are encouraged that prove fatal to the soul. Only in distrust of self and dependence on the mercy of Christ can they stand.

All who give evidence of true conversion should be encouraged to work for others. Let none turn away a soul who leaves the service of Satan for the service of Christ. When people give evidence that the Spirit of God is striving with them, present every encouragement for entering the Lord's service. "On some have compassion, making a distinction." Jude 22. Those who are wise in the wisdom that comes from God will see souls in need of help, those who have sincerely repented, but who without encouragement would hardly dare to lay hold of hope. The Lord will put it into the hearts of His servants to welcome these trembling, repentant ones to their loving fellowship. Whatever may have been their besetting sins, however low they may have fallen, when in contrition they come to Christ, He receives them. Then give them something to do for Him. If they want to help uplift others from the pit of destruction from which they themselves were rescued, give them opportunity. Bring them into association with experienced Christians, that they may gain spiritual strength. Fill their hearts and hands with work for the Master.

When light flashes into the soul, some who appeared to be most fully given to sin will become successful workers for just such sinners as they themselves once were. Through faith in Christ some will rise to high places of service and be entrusted with responsibilities in the work of saving souls. They see where their own weakness lies, they realize the depravity of their nature. They know the strength of sin, the power of evil habit. They realize their inability to overcome without the help of Christ, and their constant cry is, "I cast my helpless soul on You."

These can help others. People who have been tempted and tried, whose hope was well-nigh gone, but who were saved by hearing a message of love, can understand the science of saving souls. People whose hearts are filled with love for Christ because they themselves have been sought for by the Savior and brought back to the fold, know how to seek the lost. They can point sinners to the Lamb of God. They have given themselves without reserve to God and have been accepted in the Beloved. The hand that in weakness was held out for help has been grasped. By the ministry of such ones many prodigals will be brought to the Father.

For every soul struggling to rise from a life of sin to a life of purity, the great element of power abides in the only "'name under heaven given among men by which we must be saved.'" Acts 4:12. "'If anyone thirsts'" for restful hope, for deliverance from sinful propensities, Christ says, "'let him come to Me and drink.'" John 7:37. The only remedy for vice is the grace and power of Christ.

Good resolutions made in one's own strength avail nothing. Not all the pledges in the world will break the power of evil habit. Never will men and women practice temperance in all things until their hearts are renewed by divine grace. We cannot keep ourselves from sin for one moment. Every moment we are dependent upon God.

True reformation begins with soul cleansing. Our work for the fallen will achieve real success only as the grace of Christ reshapes the character and the soul is brought into living connection with God.

Obedience to God's Law

Christ lived a life of perfect obedience to God's law, and in this He set an example for every human being. The life that He lived in this world we are to live through His power and under His instruction.

In our work for the fallen the claims of the law of God and the need of loyalty to Him are to be impressed on mind and heart. Never fail to show that there is a marked difference between a person who serves God and one who does not serve Him. God is love, but He cannot excuse willful disregard for His commands. The enactments of His government are such that human beings do not escape the consequences of disloyalty. Only those who honor Him can He honor. Our conduct in this world decides our eternal destiny. As we sow, so we must reap. Cause will be followed by effect.

Nothing less than perfect obedience can meet the standard of God's requirement. He has not left His requirements indefinite. He has asked nothing that is not necessary in order to bring us into harmony with Him. We are to point sinners to His ideal of character and lead them to Christ, by whose grace only can this ideal be reached.

The Savior took upon Himself the infirmities of humanity and lived a sinless life that we might have no fear that because of the weakness of human nature we will be unable to overcome. Christ came to make us "partakers of the divine nature," and His life declares that humanity combined with divinity does not commit sin.

The Savior overcame to show us how we may overcome. Christ met all the temptations of Satan with the Word of God. By trusting in God's promises, He received power to obey God's commandments, and the tempter could gain no advantage. To every temptation His answer was, "It is written." So God has given us His Word by which to resist evil. Exceeding great and precious promises are ours, that by these we "may be partakers of the divine nature, having escaped the corruption that is in the world through lust." 2 Peter 1:4.

Tell the tempted one not to look at circumstances, to the weakness of self, or to the power of temptation, but to the power of God's Word. All its strength is ours. "Your word," says the psalmist, "I have hidden in my heart, that I might not sin against You." "By the word of Your lips, I have kept myself from the paths of the destroyer." Psalm 119:11; 17:4.

Talk courage to the people. Lift them up to God in prayer. Many who have been overcome by temptation are humiliated by their failures and feel that it is useless for them to approach God, but this thought is the enemy's suggestion. When they have sinned and feel that they cannot pray, tell them that then is the time to pray. They may be ashamed and deeply humbled, but as they confess their sins, He who is faithful and just will forgive their sins and cleanse them from all unrighteousness.

Nothing is apparently more helpless, yet really more invincible, than the soul that feels its nothingness and relies wholly on the merits of the Savior. By prayer, by the study of His Word, by faith in His abiding presence, the weakest of human beings may live in contact with the living Christ, and He will hold them by a hand that will never let go.

All who abide in Christ may make these precious words their own:

"I will look to the Lord;
I will wait for the God of my salvation;
My God will hear me.
Do not rejoice over me, my enemy;
When I fall, I will arise;
When I sit in darkness,
The Lord will be a light to me"
Micah 7:7, 8.
"He will again have compassion on us,
And will subdue our iniquities.
You will cast all our sins into the depths of the sea."
    Verse 19; see also Isaiah 13:12 and Psalm 68:13.

Those whom Christ has forgiven most will love Him most. These are they who in the final day will stand nearest to His throne.

"They shall see His face, and His name shall be on their foreheads." Revelation 22:4.

Help for the Unemployed and the Homeless

There are largehearted men and women who are seriously concerned about the condition of the poor and what can be done for their relief. How the unemployed and the homeless can be helped to secure the common blessings of God's providence and to live the life He intended them to live is a question to which many are earnestly endeavoring to find an answer. But there are few, even among educators and statesmen, who comprehend the causes that underlie the present state of society. Those who hold the reins of government are unable to solve the problem of poverty, pauperism, and increasing crime. They are struggling in vain to place business operations on a more secure basis.

If politicians and business leaders would give more heed to the teaching of God's Word, they would find a solution to these problems that perplex them. Much might be learned from the Old Testament in regard to the labor question and relief of the poor.

God's Plan for Israel

In God's plan for Israel every family had a home on the land with sufficient ground for cultivating. Thus were provided both the means and the incentive for a useful, industrious, and self-supporting life. And no human devising has ever improved upon that plan. The world's departure from it has caused, to a large degree, the poverty and distress that exist today.

At the settlement of Israel in Canaan, the land was divided among the whole people. The Levites only, as ministers of the sanctuary, were excepted from the equal distribution. The tribes were numbered by families, and to each family, according to its size, was apportioned an inheritance.

And although a family might for a time dispose of its possession, it could not permanently barter away the inheritance of the children. When able to redeem the land, the original owner was at liberty at any time to do so. Debts were forgiven every seventh year, and in the fiftieth, or year of jubilee, all landed property reverted to the original owner.

"'The land shall not be sold permanently,'" was the Lord's direction, "'for the land is Mine; for you are strangers and sojourners with Me. And in all the land of your possession you shall grant redemption of the land. If one of your brethren becomes poor, and has sold some of his possession, and if his kinsman-redeemer comes to redeem it, then he may redeem what his brother sold. Or if the man . . . himself becomes able to redeem it, . . . he may return to his possession. But if he is not able to have it restored to himself, then what was sold shall remain in the hand of him who bought it until the Year of Jubilee.'" Leviticus 25:23-28.

"'You shall consecrate the fiftieth year, and proclaim liberty throughout all the land to all its inhabitants. It shall be a Jubilee for you; and each of you shall return to his possession, and each of you shall return to his family.'" Verse 10.

Thus every family was secured in its possession, and a safeguard was afforded against the extremes of either wealth or poverty.

Industrial Training

In Israel, industrial training was regarded as a duty. Every father was required to teach his sons some useful trade. The greatest men in Israel were trained to industrial pursuits. A knowledge of the duties pertaining to housewifery was considered essential for every woman. And skill in these duties was regarded as an honor to women of the highest station.

Various industries were taught in the schools of the prophets, and many of the students sustained themselves by manual labor.

Consideration for the Poor

These arrangements did not, however, wholly do away with poverty. It was not God's purpose that poverty should be totally eliminated. It is one of His means for the development of character. "'The poor,'" He says, "'will never cease from the land; therefore I command you, saying, "You shall open your hand wide to your brother, to your poor and your needy, in your land."'" Deuteronomy 15:11.

"'If there is among you a poor man of your brethren, within any of the gates in your land which the Lord your God is giving you, you shall not harden your heart nor shut your hand from your poor brother, but you shall open your hand wide to him and willingly lend him sufficient for his need, whatever he needs.'" Verses 7, 8.

"'If one of your brethren becomes poor, and falls into poverty among you, then you shall help him, like a stranger or a sojourner, that he may live with you.'" Leviticus 25:35.

"'"When you reap the harvest of your land, you shall not wholly reap the corners of your field."'" "'When you reap your harvest in your field, and forget a sheaf in the field, you shall not go back to get it. . . . When you beat your olive trees, you shall not go over the boughs again. . . . When you gather the grapes of your vineyard, you shall not glean it afterward; it shall be for the stranger, the fatherless, and the widow.'" Leviticus 19:9; Deuteronomy 24:19-21.

None needed to fear that their liberality would make them poor. Obedience to God's commandments would surely result in prosperity. "'For this thing,'" God said, "'the Lord your God will bless you in all your works and in all to which you put your hand.'" "'You shall lend to many nations, but you shall not borrow; you shall reign over many nations, but they shall not reign over you.'" Deuteronomy 15:10, 6.

Business Principles

God's Word does not approve of any policy that will enrich one class by the oppression and suffering of another. It teaches us to put ourselves in the place of those with whom we are dealing in all our business transactions. We are to look out not only for our own interests but for those of others. Anyone who would take advantage of another's misfortunes in order to benefit self, or who seeks to profit through another's weakness or incompetence, is a transgressor both of the principles and of the precepts of the Word of God.

"'You shall not pervert justice due the stranger or the fatherless, nor take a widow's garment as a pledge.'" "'When you lend your brother anything, you shall not go into his house to get his pledge. You shall stand outside, and the man to whom you lend shall bring the pledge out to you. And if the man is poor, you shall not keep his pledge overnight.'" "'If you ever take your neighbor's garment as a pledge, you shall return it to him before the sun goes down. For that is his only covering. . . . What will he sleep in? And it will be that when he cries to Me, I will hear, for I am gracious.'" "'If you sell anything to your neighbor or buy from your neighbor's hand, you shall not oppress one another.'" Deuteronomy 24:17, 10-12; Exodus 22:26, 27; Leviticus 25:14.

"'You shall do no injustice in judgment, in measurement of length, weight, or volume.'" "'You shall not have in your bag differing weights, a heavy and a light. You shall not have in your house differing measures, a large and a small.'" "'You shall have honest balances, honest weights, an honest ephah, and an honest hin.'" Leviticus 19:35; Deuteronomy 25:13, 14; Leviticus 19:36.

"'Give to him who asks you, and from him who wants to borrow from you do not turn away.'" "The wicked borrows and does not repay, but the righteous shows mercy and gives." Matthew 5:42; Psalm 37:21.

"'Take counsel, execute judgment; make your shadow like the night in the middle of the day; hide the outcasts, do not betray him who escapes. Let My outcasts dwell with you, . . . be a shelter to them from the face of the spoiler.'" Isaiah 16:3, 4.

The plan of life that God gave to Israel was intended as an object lesson for the entire human family. If these principles were carried out today, what a different place this world would be!

Within the vast boundaries of nature there is still room for suffering and needy people to find a home. Within her bosom there are resources sufficient to provide them with food. Hidden in the depths of the earth are blessings for all who have the courage, will, and perseverance to gather her treasures.

Cultivating and working the soil—the employment that God appointed to Adam in Eden—opens a field in which there is opportunity for multitudes to gain a subsistence.

"Trust in the Lord, and do good;
Dwell in the land, and feed on His faithfulness."
                                        Psalm 37:3.

Thousands and tens of thousands might be working on the soil who are crowded into the cities, watching for a chance to earn a trifle. In many cases this trifle is not spent for food but is put into the coffers of the liquor seller, to obtain that which destroys soul and body.

Many look upon a regular job as drudgery, and they try to obtain a livelihood by scheming rather than by honest work. This desire to get a living without work opens the door to wretchedness, vice, and crime almost without limit.

The Inner City

In the great cities are multitudes who receive less care and consideration than are given to dumb animals. Think of the families herded together in miserable tenements, many of them in dark basements reeking with dampness and filth. In these wretched places children are born and grow up and die. They see nothing of the beauty of natural things that God has created to delight the senses and uplift the soul. Ragged and half-starved, they live amid vice and depravity, molded in character by the misery and sin that surround them. Children hear the name of God only in profanity. Foul speech, threats, and revilings fill their ears. The fumes of alcohol and tobacco, sickening stenches, moral degradation pervert their senses. Thus multitudes are trained to become criminals, enemies of a society that has abandoned them to misery and degradation.

Not all the poor in the inner city are of this class. God-fearing men and women have been brought to the depths of poverty by illness or misfortune, often through the dishonest scheming of those who live by taking advantage of others. Many who are upright and well-meaning become poor through lack of industrial training. Through ignorance they are unfitted to wrestle with the difficulties of life. Drifting into the cities, they are often unable to find employment. Surrounded by the sights and sounds of vice, they face powerful temptations. Often indiscriminately classed with the vicious and degraded, it is only by a superhuman struggle, a more-than-finite power, that they can be prevented from sinking to the same depths. Many hold fast their integrity, choosing to suffer rather than to sin. This class especially demands help, sympathy, and encouragement.

If the poor now crowded into the cities could find homes on open land, they might not only earn a livelihood but find health and happiness now unknown to them. Hard work, simple fare, close economy, often hardship and privation might be their lot, but what a blessing would be theirs in leaving the city, with its enticements to evil, its turmoil and crime, misery and foulness, for the country's quiet and peace and purity.

Many of those living in the cities have not a square foot of green grass to put their feet on. Year after year they have looked out upon filthy courts and narrow alleys, brick walls and pavements, and skies clouded with dust and smoke. If these could be taken to some farming district, with green fields, woods, hills, brooks, clear skies, and fresh, pure air, it would seem almost like heaven.

Cut off to a great degree from contact with and dependence upon other people, and separated from the world's corrupting maxims, customs, and excitements, they would come nearer to the heart of nature. God's presence would be more real to them. Many would learn the lesson of dependence upon Him. Through nature they would hear His voice speaking to their hearts of His peace and love, and mind and soul and body would respond to the healing, life-giving power.

If they ever are to become industrious and self-supporting, very many must have assistance, encouragement, and instruction. There are multitudes of poor families for whom no better missionary work could be done than to assist them in settling on the land and in learning how to make it yield them a livelihood.

The need for such help and instruction is not confined to the cities. Even in the country, with all its possibilities for a better life, multitudes of the poor are in great need. Whole communities are without education in industrial and sanitary lines. Families live in shacks, with little furniture and clothing, without tools, without books, destitute both of comforts and conveniences and of means of culture. Brutelike souls, bodies weak and ill-formed, reveal the results of evil heredity and of wrong habits. These people must be educated from the very foundation. They have led shiftless, idle, corrupt lives, and they need to be trained to correct habits.

How can they be awakened to the necessity of improvement? How can they be directed to a higher ideal of life? How can they be helped to rise? What can be done where poverty prevails and is to be contended with at every step? Certainly the work is difficult. The necessary reformation will never be made unless men and women are assisted by a power outside of themselves. It is God's purpose that the rich and the poor shall be closely bound together by ties of sympathy and helpfulness. Those who have means, talents, and capabilities are to use these gifts to bless those who are less fortunate.

Christian farmers can do real missionary work in helping the poor to find homes on the land and in teaching them how to work the soil and make it productive. Teach them how to use the implements of agriculture, how to cultivate various crops, how to plant and care for orchards.

Many who till the soil fail to secure adequate returns because of their neglect. Their orchards are not properly cared for, the crops are not put in at the right time, and a mere surface work is done in cultivating the soil. They charge their poor results to the unproductiveness of the land. False witness is often borne in condemning land that, if properly worked, would yield rich returns. The narrow plans, the little strength put forth, the little study as to the best methods, call loudly for reform.

Let proper methods be taught to all who are willing to learn. If any do not wish you to speak to them of advanced ideas, let the lessons be given silently. Keep up the culture of your own land. Drop a word to your neighbors when you can, and let the harvest be eloquent in favor of right methods. Demonstrate what can be done with the land when properly worked.

Attention should be given to the establishment of various industries so that poor families can find employment. Carpenters, blacksmiths, and indeed everyone who understands some line of useful labor should feel a responsibility to teach and help the ignorant and unemployed.

In ministry to the poor there is a wide field of service for women as well as for men. The efficient cook, the housekeeper, the seamstress, the nurse—the help of all is needed. Let the members of poor households be taught how to cook, how to make and mend their own clothing, how to nurse the sick, how to care properly for the home. Let boys and girls be thoroughly taught some useful trade or occupation.

Missionary Families

Missionary families are needed to settle in the waste places. Farmers, financiers, builders, and those who are skilled in various arts and crafts should go to neglected areas to improve the land, to establish industries, to prepare humble homes for themselves, and to help their neighbors.

The rough places of nature, the wild places, God has made attractive by placing beautiful things among the most unsightly. This is the work we are called to do. Even the desert places of the earth, where the outlook appears to be forbidding, may become as the garden of God.

"In that day the deaf shall hear the words of the book,
And the eyes of the blind shall see out of obscurity and out of darkness.
The humble also shall increase their joy in the Lord,
And the poor among men shall rejoice in the Holy One of Israel."
                                                              Isaiah 29:18, 19.

By instruction in practical matters we can often help the poor most effectively. As a rule, those who have not been trained to work do not have habits of industry, perseverance, economy, and self-denial. They do not know how to manage. Often through lack of carefulness and right judgment there is wasted that which would maintain their families in decency and comfort if it were carefully and economically used. "Much food is in the fallow ground of the poor, and for lack of justice there is waste." Proverbs 13:23.

We may give to the poor and harm them by teaching them to be dependent. Such giving encourages selfishness and helplessness. Often it leads to idleness, extravagance, and intemperance. No person who can earn his or her own livelihood has a right to depend on others. The proverb "The world owes me a living" has in it the essence of falsehood, fraud, and robbery. The world owes no one a living who is able to work.

Real charity helps people to help themselves. If they come to our door and ask for food, we should not turn them away hungry; their poverty may be the result of misfortune. But true beneficence means more than mere gifts. It means a genuine interest in the welfare of others. We should try to understand the needs of the poor and distressed, and give them the help that will benefit them most. To give thought and time and personal effort costs far more than merely to give money. But it is the truest charity.

Those who are taught to earn what they receive will more readily learn to make the most of it. And in learning to be self-reliant, they are acquiring that which will not only make them self-sustaining but enable them to help others. Teach the importance of life's duties to those who are wasting their opportunities. Show them that Bible religion never makes people idlers. Christ always encouraged industry. "'Why have you been standing here idle all day?'" He said to the indolent. "'I must work . . . while it is day; the night is coming when no one can work.'" Matthew 20:6; John 9:4.

It is the privilege of all to give to the world in their home life, in their customs and practices and order, an evidence of what the gospel can do for those who obey it. Christ came to our world to give us an example of what we may become. He expects His followers to be models of correctness in all the relations of life. He desires the divine touch to be seen upon outward things.

Our own homes and surroundings should be object lessons, teaching ways of improvement, so that industry, cleanliness, taste, and refinement may take the place of idleness, uncleanness, coarseness, and disorder. By our lives and example we can help others to discern that which is repulsive in their character or their surroundings, and with Christian courtesy we may encourage improvement. As we manifest an interest in them, we shall find opportunity to teach them how to put their energies to the best use.

Hope and Courage

We can do nothing without courage and perseverance. Speak words of hope and courage to the poor and the disheartened. If need be, give tangible proof of your interest by helping them when they face difficult situations. Those who have had many advantages should remember that they themselves still err in many things, and that it is painful to them when their errors are pointed out and they are shown an inspiring pattern of what they should be. Remember that kindness will accomplish more than censure. As you try to teach others, let them see that you wish them to reach the highest standard, and that you are ready to give them help. If in some things they fail, do not be quick to condemn them.

Simplicity, self-denial, economy—lessons essential for the poor to learn—often seem to them difficult and unwelcome. The example and spirit of the world is constantly exciting and fostering pride, love of display, self-indulgence, extravagance, and idleness. These evils bring thousands to poverty and prevent thousands more from rising out of degradation and wretchedness. Christians are to encourage the poor to resist these influences.

Jesus came to this world in humility. He was of lowly birth. Though He was the Majesty of heaven, the King of glory, the Commander of all the angel host, He humbled Himself to accept humanity, and then He chose a life of poverty and humiliation. He had no opportunities that today's poor do not have. Toil, hardship, and privation were part of His everyday experience. "'Foxes have holes,'" He said, "'and birds of the air have nests, but the Son of Man has nowhere to lay His head.'" Luke 9:58.

Jesus did not seek admiration or applause from the people. He commanded no army. He ruled no earthly kingdom. He did not court the favor of the wealthy and honored of the world. He did not claim a position among the leaders of the nation. He lived among the lowly. He repudiated the artificial distinctions of society. He ignored the aristocracy of birth, wealth, talent, learning, rank.

He was the Prince of heaven, yet He did not choose His disciples from among the learned lawyers, rulers, scribes, or Pharisees. He passed these by, because they prided themselves on their learning and position. They were fixed in their traditions and superstitions. He who could read all hearts chose humble fishermen who were willing to be taught. He ate with publicans and sinners and mingled with the common people, not to become low and earthly with them but by precept and example to present to them right principles and to uplift them from their earthliness and debasement.

Jesus sought to correct the world's false standard of how to judge the value of people. He took His position with the poor so that He might lift from poverty the stigma that the world had attached to it. He has stripped from it forever the reproach of scorn by blessing the poor, the inheritors of God's kingdom. He points us to the path He trod, saying, "'If anyone desires to come after Me, let him deny himself, and take up his cross daily, and follow Me.'" Luke 9:23.

Christian workers are to meet the people where they are and educate them, not in pride but in character building. Teach them how Christ worked and denied Himself. Help them to learn from Him the lessons of self-denial and sacrifice. Teach them to beware of self-indulgence in conforming to fashion. Life is too valuable, too full of solemn, sacred responsibilities, to be wasted in pleasing self.

Life's Best Things

Men and women have hardly begun to understand the true object of life. They are attracted by glitter and show. They are ambitious for worldly preeminence. To this the true aims of life are sacrificed. Life's best things—simplicity, honesty, truthfulness, purity, integrity—cannot be bought or sold. They are as free to the ignorant as to the educated, to the humble worker as to the honored statesman. For everyone God has provided pleasure that may be enjoyed by rich and poor alike—the pleasure found in cultivating pureness of thought and unselfishness of action, the pleasure that comes from speaking sympathizing words and doing kindly deeds. From those who perform such service, the light of Christ shines to brighten lives darkened by many shadows.

While helping the poor in temporal things, keep always in view their spiritual needs. Let your own life testify to the Savior's keeping power. Let your character reveal the high standard to which all may attain. Teach the gospel in simple object lessons. Let everything with which you have to do be a lesson in character building.

In the humble round of toil, the very weakest, the most obscure, may be workers together with God and may have the comfort of His presence and sustaining grace. They are not to weary themselves with busy anxieties and needless cares. Let them work on from day to day, accomplishing faithfully the task that God's providence assigns, and He will care for them. Through the apostle Paul He says:

"Be anxious for nothing, but in everything by prayer and supplication, with thanksgiving, let your requests be made known to God; and the peace of God, which surpasses all understanding, will guard your hearts and minds through Christ Jesus." Philippians 4:6, 7.

The Lord's care is over all His creatures. He loves them all and makes no difference, except that He has the most tender pity for those who are called to bear life's heaviest burdens. God's children must meet trials and difficulties. But they should accept their lot with a cheerful spirit, remembering that for all that the world neglects to bestow, God Himself will make up to them in the best of favors.

It is when we come into difficult places that He reveals His power and wisdom in answer to humble prayer. Have confidence in Him as a prayer-hearing, prayer-answering God. He will reveal Himself to you as One who can help in every emergency. He who created us, who gave us wonderful physical, mental, and spiritual faculties, will not withhold that which is necessary to sustain the life He has given. He who has given us His word—the leaves of the tree of life—will not withhold from us a knowledge of how to provide food for His needy children.

How can wisdom be obtained by one who holds the plow and drives the oxen? By seeking her as silver, and searching for her as for hid treasure. "For He instructs him in right judgment, his God teaches him." Isaiah 28:26. "This also comes from the Lord of hosts, who is wonderful in counsel and excellent in guidance." Verse 29.

He who taught Adam and Eve in Eden how to tend the garden desires to instruct us today. There is wisdom for one who drives the plow and sows the seed. For those who trust and obey Him, God will open ways of advance. Let them move forward courageously, trusting in Him to supply their needs according to the riches of His goodness.

He who fed the multitude with five loaves and two small fish is able today to give us the fruit of our labor. He who said to the fishers of Galilee, "Let down your nets for a catch," and who, as they obeyed, filled their nets till they broke, desires His people to see in this an evidence of what He will do for them today. The God who in the wilderness gave the children of Israel manna from heaven still lives and reigns. He will guide His people and give skill and understanding in the work they are called to do. He will give wisdom to those who strive to do their duty conscientiously and intelligently. He who owns the world is rich in resources and will bless everyone who is seeking to bless others.

We need to look heavenward in faith. We are not to be discouraged because of apparent failure, nor should we be disheartened by delay. We should work cheerfully, hopefully, gratefully, believing that the earth holds in her bosom rich treasures for the faithful worker to garner, stores richer than gold or silver. The mountains and hills are changing, the earth is growing old like a garment, but the blessing of God, which spreads for His people a table in the wilderness, will never cease.

C h a p t e r   13

The
Helpless Poor

When all has been done that can be done in helping the poor to help themselves, there still remain the widow, the fatherless, the aged, the helpless, and the sick, who need sympathy and care. Never should these be neglected. God Himself has committed them to the mercy, love, and tender care of all whom He has made His stewards.

"As we have opportunity, let us do good to all, especially to those who are of the household of faith." Galatians 6:10.

In a special sense, Christ has laid upon His church the duty of caring for the needy among its own members. He permits His poor to be in every church. They are always to be among us, and He places upon the members of the church a personal responsibility to care for them.

As the members of a true family care for one another, ministering to the sick, supporting the weak, teaching the ignorant, training the inexperienced, so is "the household of faith" to care for its needy and helpless ones. Upon no consideration are these to be passed by.

Widows and Orphans
The widow and the fatherless are the objects of the Lord's special care.

"A father of the fatherless, a defender of widows,
Is God in His holy habitation."
"'Your Maker is your husband,
The Lord of hosts is His name;

And your Redeemer is the Holy One of Israel;
He is called the God of the whole earth.'"

"'Leave your fatherless children,
I will preserve them alive;
And let your widows trust in Me.'"
          Psalm 68:5; Isaiah 54:5; Jeremiah 49:11.

Many a father, when called upon to part from his loved ones, has died resting in faith upon God's promise to care for them. The Lord provides for the widow and the fatherless, not by a miracle in sending manna from heaven, not by sending ravens to bring them food, but by a miracle upon human hearts, expelling selfishness and unsealing the fountains of Christlike love. He commits the afflicted and bereaved ones to His followers as a precious trust. They have the very strongest claim upon our sympathy.

In homes supplied with life's comforts, in granaries filled with the yield of abundant harvests, in warehouses stocked with the products of the loom, and vaults stored with gold and silver, God has supplied means for the sustenance of these needy ones. He calls upon us to be channels of His bounty.

Many a widowed mother with her fatherless children is bravely striving to bear her double burden, often working far beyond her strength in order to keep her little ones with her and to provide for their needs. She has little time for their training and instruction, little opportunity to surround them with influences that would brighten their lives. She needs encouragement, sympathy, and tangible help.

God calls upon us to supply to these children, so far as we can, what they lack from a father's care. Instead of standing aloof, complaining of their faults and of the trouble they may cause, help them in every way possible. Seek to aid the careworn mother. Lighten her burdens.

Then there are the multitudes of children who have been wholly deprived of the guidance of parents and the subduing influence of a Christian home. Let Christians open their hearts and homes to these helpless ones. The work that God has committed to them as an individual duty should not be turned over to some benevolent institution or left to the chances of the world's charity. If the children have no relatives able to give them care, the members of the church should provide homes for them. He who created us planned that we should be associated in families, and a child's nature will develop best in the loving atmosphere of a Christian home.

Many who have no children of their own could do a good work in caring for the children of others. Instead of giving attention to pets, lavishing affection upon animals, let them give their attention to little children, whose characters they may fashion after the divine similitude. Place your love upon the homeless members of the human family. See how many of these children you can bring up in the nurture and admonition of the Lord. Christians who do this will be greatly benefited themselves.

The Elderly

Older people also need the helpful influences of the family. If they no longer have their own home, the blessings and influences thus lost can best be made up in the home of fellow Christians. Encouraging them to share in the interests and occupations of the household will help them feel that they are still useful. Make them feel that their help is valued, that there is something yet for them to do in ministering to others, and it will cheer their hearts and give interest to their lives.

So far as possible, those who are near the end of life's journey should remain among friends and familiar associations. Let them worship among those whom they have known and loved. Let them be cared for by loving and tender hands.

Whenever the members of a family are able to do so, they should count it a privilege to minister to their own kindred. When this cannot be, the work belongs to the church, and it should be accepted both as a privilege and as a duty. All who possess Christ's spirit will have a tender regard for the feeble and the elderly.

The presence in our homes of one of these helpless ones is a precious opportunity to cooperate with Christ in His ministry of mercy and to develop traits of character like His. There is a blessing for both old and young in associating together. The young may bring sunshine into the hearts and lives of the aged. Those whose hold on life is weakening need the benefit of contact with the hopefulness and buoyancy of youth. And the young may be helped by the wisdom and experience of the old. Above all, they need to learn the lesson of unselfish ministry. The presence of a person in need of sympathy and forbearance and self-sacrificing love would be to many a household a priceless blessing. It would sweeten and refine the home life and call forth in old and young those Christlike graces that would make them beautiful with a divine beauty and rich in heaven's imperishable treasure.

A Test of Character

"'You have the poor with you always,'" Christ said, "'and whenever you wish you may do them good.'" "Pure and undefiled religion before God and the Father is this: to visit orphans and widows in their trouble, and to keep oneself unspotted from the world." Mark 14:7; James 1:27.

Christ tests His professed followers by placing among them the helpless and the poor, to be dependent upon their care. Our love and service for His needy children prove the genuineness of our love for Him. To neglect them is to declare ourselves false disciples, strangers to Christ and His love.

If we were to do all we could in providing homes in families for orphans, many others would still require care. Many have received an inheritance of evil. They are unpromising, unattractive, perverse, but they are the purchase of the blood of Christ, and in His sight are just as precious as are our own little ones. Unless a helping hand is held out to them, they will grow up in ignorance and drift into vice and crime. Many of these children could be rescued through the work of orphanages.

Such institutions, to be most effective, should be modeled as closely as possible after the plan of a Christian home. Instead of large establishments, bringing great numbers together, there should be small institutions in a number of places. Instead of being in or near some town or large city, they should be in the country, where land can be secured for cultivation and the children can be brought into contact with nature and can have the benefits of industrial training.

Those in charge of such a home should be men and women who are largehearted, cultured, and self-sacrificing, men and women who undertake the work from love to Christ and who train the children for Him. Under such care many homeless and neglected ones may be prepared to become useful members of society, an honor to Christ, and a help to others.

Many despise economy, equating it with stinginess and narrowness. But economy is consistent with the broadest liberality. Indeed, without economy there can be no true liberality. We are to save that we may give.

No one can practice real benevolence without self-denial. Only by a life of simplicity, self-denial, and close economy is it possible for us to accomplish the work appointed us as Christ's representatives. Pride and worldly ambition must be put out of our hearts. In all our work the principle of unselfishness revealed in Christ's life is to be carried out. Upon the walls of our homes, the pictures, and the furnishings, we are to read, "Bring to your house the poor who are cast out." On our wardrobes we are to see written, as with the finger of God, "Clothe the naked." In the dining room, on the table laden with abundant food, we should see traced, "Is it not to share your bread with the hungry?" Isaiah 58:7.

A thousand doors of usefulness are open before us. Often we lament the scanty resources available, but if Christians were thoroughly in earnest, they could multiply the resources a thousandfold. It is selfishness, self-indulgence, that bars the way to our usefulness.

How much money is expended for things that are mere idols, things that engross thought and time and strength that should be put to a higher use! How much means is wasted on expensive houses and furniture, on selfish pleasures, luxurious and unwholesome food, hurtful indulgences!

How much is squandered on gifts that benefit no one! For things that are needless, often harmful, professed Christians are today spending more, many times more, than they spend in seeking to rescue souls from the tempter.

Many who profess to be Christians spend so much on dress that they have nothing to spare for the needs of others. They think they must have costly ornaments and expensive clothing regardless of the needs of those who have difficulty providing themselves with even the plainest clothing.

My sisters, if you would bring your manner of dressing into conformity with the rules given in the Bible, you would have an abundance with which to help your poorer sisters. You would have not only means but time. Often this is most needed. There are many whom you might help with your suggestions, your tact and skill. Show them how to dress simply and yet tastefully. Many a woman remains away from the house of God because her shabby, ill-fitting garments are in such striking contrast to the dress of others. Many a sensitive spirit cherishes a sense of bitter humiliation and injustice because of this contrast. And because of it many are led to doubt the reality of religion and to harden their hearts against the gospel.

Christ commands us, "Gather up the fragments that remain, that nothing be lost." While thousands are every day perishing from famine, bloodshed, fire, and plague, everyone who loves people should see that nothing is wasted, that nothing is needlessly expended that might benefit a human being.

It is wrong to waste our time, wrong to waste our thoughts. We lose every moment that we devote to self-seeking. If every moment were valued and rightly employed, we would have time for everything that we need to do for ourselves or for the world. In the expenditure of money, in the use of time, strength, opportunities, let every Christian look to God for guidance. "If any of you lacks wisdom, let him ask of God, who gives to all liberally and without reproach, and it will be given to him." James 1:5.

" 'Do good, and lend, hoping for nothing in return; and your reward will be great, and you will be sons of the Highest. For He is kind to the unthankful and evil.' " Luke 6:35.

"He who hides his eyes will have many curses," but "he who gives to the poor will not lack." Proverbs 28:27.

" 'Give, and it will be given to you: good measure, pressed down, shaken together, and running over will be put into your bosom.' " Luke 6:38.

Chapter 14

Ministry
to the Rich

Cornelius, the Roman centurion, was a man of wealth and noble birth. His position was one of trust and honor. Though a heathen by birth, training, and education, through contact with the Jews he had gained a knowledge of the true God, and he worshiped Him, showing the sincerity of his faith by compassion to the poor. He gave "alms generously to the people, and prayed to God always." Acts 10:2.

But Cornelius had no knowledge of the gospel as revealed in the life and death of Christ. So God sent a message direct from heaven to him and also directed the apostle Peter to visit and instruct him. Cornelius was not united with the Jewish church and would have been looked upon by the rabbis as a heathen and unclean. But God read the sincerity of his heart and sent messengers from His throne to unite with His servant on earth in teaching the gospel to this officer of Rome.

So today God is seeking for souls among the high as well as the low. There are many like Cornelius, men and women whom He desires to connect with His church. Their sympathies are with the Lord's people. But the ties that bind them to the world hold them firmly. It requires moral courage for these people to take their position with the lowly ones. Special effort should be made for these souls who are in so great danger because of their responsibilities and associations.

Much is said concerning our duty to the neglected poor, but should not some attention be given to the neglected rich? Many look upon this class as hopeless, and they do little to open the eyes of those who, blinded and dazed by the glitter of earthly glory, have left eternity out of their reckoning. Thousands of wealthy people have gone to their graves unwarned. But indifferent as they may appear, many among the rich are soul-burdened. "He who loves silver will not be satisfied with silver; nor he who loves abundance, with increase." He that says to fine gold, "'"You are my confidence,"'" has "'denied God who is above.'" "None of them can by any means redeem his brother, nor give to God a ransom for him—for the redemption of their souls is costly, and it shall cease forever." Ecclesiastes 5:10; Job 31:24, 28; Psalm 49:7, 8.

Riches and worldly honor cannot satisfy the soul. Many among the rich are longing for some divine assurance, some spiritual hope. Many long for something that will bring to an end the monotony of their aimless lives. Many in official life feel their need of something that they do not have. Few among them go to church, for they feel that they receive little benefit. The teaching they hear does not touch the heart. Shall we make no personal appeal to them?

Among the victims of want and sin are some who were once in possession of wealth. Men and women of different vocations and different stations in life have been overcome by the pollutions of the world, by the use of strong drink, by the indulgence of lust and have fallen under temptation. While these fallen ones demand pity and help, should not some attention be given to those who have not yet descended to these depths but who are setting their feet in the same path?

Thousands in positions of trust and honor are indulging habits that mean ruin to soul and body. Ministers of the gospel, statesmen, authors, men and women of wealth and talent, people of vast business capacity and power for usefulness, are in deadly peril because they do not see the necessity of self-control in all things. They need to have their attention called to the principles of temperance, not in a narrow or arbitrary way, but in the light of God's great purpose for humanity. If the principles of true temperance were brought before them, very many of the higher classes would recognize their value and give them a hearty acceptance.

Show these persons the result of harmful indulgences in lessening physical, mental, and moral power. Help them to realize their respon-sibility as stewards of God's gifts. Show them the good they could do with the money they now spend for that which does them only harm. Urge them to stop using liquor, tobacco, and similar products, and ask that the money they would otherwise spend for these indulgences be devoted to relief of the sick poor or for the training of children and youth for usefulness in the world. Many would respond to such an appeal.

The Dangers of Prosperity

There is another danger to which the wealthy are especially exposed, and here also is a field for the medical missionary. Multitudes who are prosperous in the world and who never stoop to the common forms of vice are yet brought to destruction through the love of riches. The cup most difficult to carry is not the cup that is empty but the cup that is full to the brim. It is this that needs to be most carefully balanced. Affliction and adversity bring disappointment and sorrow, but it is prosperity that is most dangerous to spiritual life.

Those who are suffering reverses are represented by the bush that Moses saw in the desert, which, though burning, was not consumed. The Angel of the Lord was in the midst of the bush. So in deprivation and affliction the brightness of the presence of the Unseen is with us to comfort and sustain. Often prayer is solicited for those who are suffering from illness or adversity, but our prayers are most needed by the people entrusted with prosperity and influence.

In the valley of humiliation, where souls feel their need and depend on God to guide their steps, there is comparative safety. But people who stand, as it were, on a lofty pinnacle, and who, because of their position, are supposed to possess great wisdom—these are in greatest peril. Unless they make God their dependence, they will surely fall.

The Bible condemns no one for being rich if the riches have been acquired honestly. Not money, but the love of money, is the root of all evil. It is God who gives people power to get wealth, and in the hands of one who acts as God's steward, using the means unselfishly, wealth is a blessing, both to its possessor and to the world. But many, absorbed in their interest in worldly treasures, become insensible to the claims of God and the needs of others. They regard their wealth as a means of glorifying themselves. They add house to house, and land to land; they fill their homes with luxuries, while all about them are human beings in misery and crime, in disease and death. Those who thus give their lives to self-serving are developing in themselves not the attributes of God but the attributes of the wicked one.

These people need the gospel. They need to have their eyes turned from the vanity of material things to behold the preciousness of the enduring riches. They need to learn the joy of giving, the blessedness of being co-workers with God.

The Lord bids us, "Command those who are rich in this present age" not to trust "in uncertain riches but in the living God, who gives us richly all things to enjoy. Let them do good, that they be rich in good works, ready to give, willing to share, storing up for themselves a good foundation for the time to come, that they may lay hold on eternal life." 1 Timothy 6:17-19.

It is not by casual, accidental touch that wealthy, world-loving, world-worshiping people will be drawn to Christ. Often these are the most difficult to get access to. Personal effort must be put forth for them by men and women imbued with the missionary spirit, those who will not fail or be discouraged.

Working for the Higher Classes

Some are especially fitted to work for the higher classes. These should seek wisdom from God to know how to reach these persons, not to have merely a casual acquaintance with them, but by personal effort and living faith to awaken them to the needs of the soul, to lead them to a knowledge of the truth as it is in Jesus.

Many suppose that in order to reach the higher classes, a manner of life and method of work must be adopted that will be suited to their fastidious tastes. An appearance of wealth, costly buildings, stylish dress, expensive cars and surroundings, conformity to worldly customs, the artificial polish of fashionable society, classical culture, the graces of oratory are thought to be essential. This is an error. The way of worldly policy is not God's way of reaching the higher classes. That which will reach them effectually is a consistent, unselfish presentation of the gospel of Christ.

The experience of the apostle Paul in meeting the philosophers of Athens has a lesson for us. In presenting the gospel before the court of the Areopagus, Paul met logic with logic, science with science, philosophy with philosophy. The wisest of his hearers were astonished and silenced. His words could not be controverted. But the effort bore little fruit. Few were led to accept the gospel. Henceforth Paul adopted a different method of work. He avoided elaborate arguments and discussion of theories, and in simplicity pointed men and women to Christ as the Savior of sinners.

Writing to the Corinthians of his work among them, he said: "I, brethren, when I came to you, did not come with excellence of speech or of wisdom declaring to you the testimony of God. For I determined not to know anything among you except Jesus Christ and Him crucified. . . . My speech and my preaching were not with persuasive words of human wisdom, but in demonstration of the Spirit and of power, that your faith should not be in the wisdom of men but in the power of God." 1 Corinthians 2:1-5.

Again, in his letter to the Romans, he says: "I am not ashamed of the gospel of Christ, for it is the power of God to salvation for everyone who believes, for the Jew first and also for the Greek." Romans 1:16.

Let those who work for the higher classes bear themselves with true dignity, remembering that angels are their companions. Let them keep the treasure house of mind and heart filled with "It is written." Hang in memory's hall the precious words of Christ. They are to be valued far above gold or silver.

Christ said that it is easier for a camel to go through the eye of a needle than for the rich to enter the kingdom of God. In the work for this class many discouragements will be presented, many heartsickening revelations will be made. But all things are possible with God. He can and will work through human agencies upon the minds of people whose lives have been devoted to money getting.

There are miracles to be wrought in genuine conversion, miracles that are not now discerned. The greatest men and women of the earth are not beyond the power of a wonder-working God. If those who are workers together with Him will do their duty bravely and faithfully, God will convert people who occupy responsible places, persons of intellect and influence. Through the power of the Holy Spirit, many will be led to accept the divine principles.

When it is made plain to them that the Lord expects them as His representatives to relieve suffering humanity, many will respond and will give of their means and their sympathies for the benefit of the poor. As their minds are thus drawn away from their selfish interests, many will surrender themselves to Christ. With their talents of influence and means they will gladly unite in the work of beneficence with the humble missionary who was God's agent in their conversion. By a right use of their earthly treasures they will lay up for themselves "treasures in heaven, where neither moth nor rust destroys and where thieves do not break in and steal."

When converted to Christ, many will become agents in the hand of God to work for others of their own class. They will feel that the gospel has been committed to them so that they can give it to those who have made this world their all. Time and money will be consecrated to God, talent and influence will be devoted to the work of winning souls to Christ.

Only eternity will reveal what has been accomplished by this kind of ministry—how many souls, sick with doubt and tired of worldliness and unrest, have been brought to the great Restorer, who longs to save to the uttermost all who come to Him. Christ is a risen Savior, and there is healing in His wings.

The Care of the Sick

C h a p t e r   15

In the
Sickroom

Those who minister to the sick should understand the importance of careful attention to the laws of health. Nowhere is obedience to these laws more important than in the sickroom. Nowhere does so much depend upon faithfulness in little things on the part of caregivers. In cases of serious illness, a little neglect, a slight inattention to a patient's special needs or dangers, the manifestation of fear, excitement, or petulance, even a lack of sympathy may tip the scale that is balancing life against death and send to the grave a patient who otherwise might have recovered.

The efficiency of nurses depends, to a great degree, upon physical vigor. The better the health, the better will they be able to endure the strain of attendance upon the sick, and the more successfully can they perform their duties. Those who care for the sick at home should give special attention to diet, cleanliness, fresh air, and exercise. The same kind of carefulness on the part of the family will enable them also to endure the extra burdens brought upon them and will help prevent them from contracting disease.

Where the illness is serious, requiring round-the-clock nursing, the work should be shared by at least two efficient nurses, so that each may have opportunity for rest and for exercise in the open air. This is especially important in some homes where it is difficult to secure an abundance of fresh air in the sickroom. Sometimes, because the importance of fresh air is not understood, ventilation is restricted, and the lives of both patient and caregiver are endangered.

If proper precautions are observed, the disease need not be taken by others. Let the habits be correct, and by cleanliness and proper ventilation keep the sickroom free from poisonous elements. Under such conditions, the sick are much more likely to recover, and in most cases neither caregivers nor the members of the family will contract the disease.

Sunlight, Ventilation, and Temperature

To afford the most favorable conditions for recovery, the patient should be placed in a large, sunny room, with opportunity for thorough ventilation. Many houses have no special provision for proper ventilation, and to secure it is difficult, but every possible effort should be made to arrange the sickroom so that a current of fresh air can pass through it night and day.

So far as possible an even temperature should be maintained in the sickroom. A thermometer should be consulted. Those who have the care of the sick, being often deprived of sleep or awakened in the night to attend to the patient, are likely to feel chilly and are not good judges of a healthful temperature.

Diet

An important part of the duty of those who attend the sick is to supervise the patient's diet. The patient should not be allowed to become unduly weak through lack of nourishment, nor should the enfeebled digestive powers be overtaxed. Care should be taken to prepare and serve food that will be palatable, but wise judgment should be used in adapting it to the needs of the patient, both in quantity and quality. In times of convalescence especially, when the appetite is keen, before the digestive organs have recovered strength, there is great danger of injury from errors in diet.

Duties of Attendants

Nurses, and all who have to do with the sickroom, should be cheerful, calm, and self-possessed. All hurry, excitement, or confusion should be avoided. Doors should be opened and shut with care, and the whole household be kept quiet. In cases of fever, special care is needed when the crisis comes and the fever is passing away. Then constant watching is often necessary. Ignorance, forgetfulness, and recklessness have caused the death of many who might have lived had they received proper care from judicious, thoughtful nurses.

Visiting the Sick

It is misdirected kindness, a false idea of courtesy, that leads to much visiting of the sick. Those who are very ill should not have visitors. The excitement connected with receiving callers wearies patients at a time when they are in the greatest need of quiet, undisturbed rest.

To convalescents or patients suffering from chronic disease, it is often a pleasure and a benefit to know that they are kindly remembered, but this assurance conveyed by a message of sympathy or by some little gift will often accomplish more than a personal visit, and without danger of harm.

Institutional Nursing

In sanitariums and hospitals, where nurses are constantly associated with large numbers of sick people, it requires a decided effort to be always pleasant and cheerful and show thoughtful consideration in every word and act. In these institutions it is of the utmost importance that nurses strive to do their work wisely and well. They need ever to remember that in the discharge of their daily duties they are serving the Lord Christ.

The sick need to have wise words spoken to them. Nurses should study the Bible daily that they may be able to speak words that will enlighten and help the suffering. Angels of God are in the rooms where suffering ones are being ministered to, and the atmosphere surrounding the soul of the one giving treatment should be pure and fragrant. Physicians and nurses are to cherish the principles of Christ. In their lives His virtues are to be seen. Then, by what they do and say, they will draw the sick to the Savior.

The Christian nurse, while administering treatment for the restoration of health, will pleasantly and successfully draw the mind of the patient to Christ, the healer of the soul as well as of the body. The thoughts presented, here a little and there a little, will have their influence. The older nurses should lose no favorable opportunity of calling the attention of the sick to Christ. They should be ever ready to blend spiritual healing with physical healing.

In the kindest and tenderest manner, nurses are to teach that patients who would be healed must cease to transgress the law of God. They must cease to choose a life of sin. God cannot bless those who continue to bring upon themselves disease and suffering by willful violation of the laws of heaven. But Christ, through the Holy Spirit, comes as a healing power to those who cease to do evil and learn to do well.

Those who have no love for God will work constantly against the best interests of soul and body. But those who awake to the importance of living in obedience to God in this present evil world will be willing to separate from every wrong habit. Gratitude and love will fill their hearts. They know that Christ is their friend. In many cases the realization that they have such a friend means more to the suffering ones in their recovery from sickness than the best treatment that can be given. But both lines of ministry are essential. They are to go hand in hand.

Prayer
for the Sick

The Scripture says that "men always ought to pray and not lose heart" Luke 18:1. If ever there is a time when people feel their need of prayer, it is when strength fails and life itself seems slipping from their grasp. Often those who are in health forget the wonderful mercies extended to them day by day, year after year, and they render no tribute of praise to God for His benefits. But when sickness comes, God is remembered. When human strength fails, people feel their need of divine help. And never does our merciful God turn from the soul that in sincerity seeks Him for help. He is our refuge in sickness as in health.

"As a father pities his children,
So the Lord pities those who fear Him.
For He knows our frame;
He remembers that we are dust."
          Psalm 103:13, 14.

"Because of their transgression,
And because of their iniquities, [people] were afflicted.
Their soul abhorred all manner of food,
And they drew near to the gates of death.
Then they cried out to the Lord in their trouble,
And He saved them out of their distresses.
He sent His word and healed them,

And delivered them from their destructions."
Psalm 107:17-20.

God is just as willing to restore the sick to health now as when the Holy Spirit spoke these words through the psalmist. And Christ is the same compassionate Physician now that He was during His earthly ministry. In Him there is healing balm for every disease, restoring power for every infirmity. His disciples in this time are to pray for the sick as verily as the disciples of old prayed. And recoveries will follow, for "the prayer of faith will save the sick." We have the Holy Spirit's power, the calm assurance of faith, that can claim God's promises.

The Lord's promise, "'They will lay hands on the sick, and they will recover'" (Mark 16:18), is just as trustworthy now as in the days of the apostles. It presents the privilege of God's children, and our faith should lay hold of all that it embraces. Christ's servants are the channel of His working, and through them He desires to exercise His healing power. It is our work to present the sick and suffering to God in the arms of our faith. We should teach them to believe in the Great Healer.

The Savior would have us encourage the sick, the hopeless, the afflicted, to take hold upon His strength. Through faith and prayer the sickroom may be transformed into a Bethel. In word and deed, physicians and nurses may say, so plainly that it cannot be misunderstood, "God is in this place" to save, and not to destroy. Christ desires to manifest His presence in the sickroom, filling the hearts of physicians and nurses with the sweetness of His love. If the life of those who attend the sick is such that Christ can go with them to the bedside of the patient, there will come to the sick the conviction that the compassionate Savior is present, and this conviction will itself do much for the healing of both soul and body.

God hears prayer. Christ has said, "'If you ask anything in My name, I will do it.'" Again He says, "'If anyone serves Me, him My Father will honor.'" John 14:14; 12:26. If we live according to His Word, every precious promise He has given will be fulfilled to us. We are undeserving of His mercy, but as we give ourselves to Him, He receives us. He will work for and through those who follow Him.

But only as we live in obedience to His Word can we claim the fulfillment of His promises. The psalmist says, "If I regard iniquity in my heart, the LORD will not hear." Psalm 66:18. If we render to Him only a partial, halfhearted obedience, His promises will not be fulfilled to us.

In the Word of God we have instruction relative to special prayer for the recovery of the sick. The offering of such prayer is a most solemn act and should not be entered upon without careful consideration. In many cases of prayer for healing of the sick, that which is called faith is nothing less than presumption.

Abandon Unhealthful Practices

Many persons bring disease upon themselves by self-indulgence. They have not lived in accordance with natural law or the principles of strict purity. Others have disregarded the laws of health in their habits of eating and drinking, dressing, or working. Often some form of vice is the cause of feebleness of mind or body. If these persons were to gain the blessing of health, many of them would continue to pursue the same course of heedless transgression of God's natural and spiritual laws. They would reason that if God heals them in answer to prayer, they are at liberty to continue their unhealthful practices and to indulge perverted appetite. If God were to work a miracle in restoring these persons to health, He would be encouraging sin.

It is labor lost to teach people to look to God as a healer of their infirmities unless they are taught also to lay aside unhealthful practices. In order to receive His blessing in answer to prayer, they must cease to do evil and learn to do well. Their surroundings must be sanitary, their habits of life correct. They must live in harmony with the law of God, both natural and spiritual.

Confession of Sin

To those who desire prayer for restoration to health, it should be made plain that the violation of God's law, either natural or spiritual, is sin, and that in order for them to receive His blessing, sin must be confessed and forsaken.

The Scripture bids us, "Confess your trespasses to one another, and pray for one another, that you may be healed." James 5:16. To the one asking for prayer, let thoughts like these be presented: "We cannot read the heart or know the secrets of your life. These are known only to yourself and to God. If you repent of your sins, it is your duty to confess them." Sin of a private character is to be confessed to Christ, the only mediator between God and man. For "if anyone sins, we have an Advocate with the Father, Jesus Christ the righteous." 1 John 2:1. Every sin is an offense against God and is to be confessed to Him through Christ.

Every open sin should be as openly confessed. Wrong done to a fellow being should be made right with the one who has been offended. If any who are seeking health have been guilty of evilspeaking, if they have sowed discord in the home, the neighborhood, or the church and have stirred up alienation and dissension, if by any wrong practice they have led others into sin, these things should be confessed before God and before those who have been offended. "If we confess our sins, He is faithful and just to forgive us our sins and to cleanse us from all unrighteousness." 1 John 1:9.

When wrongs have been righted, we may present the needs of the sick to the Lord in calm faith, as His Spirit may indicate. He knows each person by name and cares for each as if there were not another upon the earth for whom He gave His beloved Son. Because God's love is so great and so unfailing, the sick should be encouraged to trust in Him and be cheerful. To be anxious about themselves tends to cause weakness and disease. If they will rise above depression and gloom, their prospect of recovery will be better, for "the eye of the Lord is on those . . . who hope in His mercy." Psalm 33:18.

God Knows Best

In prayer for the sick it should be remembered that "we do not know what we should pray for as we ought." Romans 8:26. We do not know whether the blessing we desire will be best. Therefore our prayers should include this thought: "Lord, you know every secret of the soul. You are acquainted with these persons. Jesus, their Advocate, gave His life for them. His love for them is greater than ours can possibly be. If, therefore, it is for Your glory and the good of the afflicted ones, we ask, in the name of Jesus, that they may be restored to health. If it is not Your will that they may be restored, we ask that Your grace may comfort and Your presence sustain them in their sufferings."

God knows the end from the beginning. He is acquainted with the hearts of all human beings. He reads every secret of the soul. He knows whether those for whom prayer is offered would be able to endure the trials that would come upon them should they live. He knows whether their lives would be a blessing or a curse to themselves and to the world. This is one reason why, while presenting our petitions with earnestness, we should say, "Nevertheless not my will, but Yours, be done." Luke 22:42. Jesus added these words of submission to the wisdom and will of God when in the Garden of Gethsemane He pleaded, "O My Father, if it is possible, let this cup pass from Me." Matthew 26:39. And if they were appropriate for Him, the Son of God, how much more appropriate are they on the lips of finite, erring mortals!

The consistent course is to commit our desires to our all-wise heavenly Father, and then, in perfect confidence, trust all to Him. We know that God hears us if we ask according to His will. But to press our petitions without a submissive spirit is not right. Our prayers must take the form, not of command, but of intercession.

There are cases where God works decidedly by His divine power in the restoration of health. But not all the sick are healed. Many are laid away to sleep in Jesus. John on the Isle of Patmos was bidden to write: " ' "Blessed are the dead who die in the Lord from now on." ' 'Yes,' says the Spirit, 'that they may rest from their labors, and their works follow them.'" Revelation 14:13. From this we see that if persons are not raised to health, they should not on this account be judged as lacking in faith.

We all desire immediate and direct answers to our prayers and are tempted to become discouraged when the answer is delayed or comes in an unlooked-for form. But God is too wise and too good to answer our prayers always at just the time and in just the way we desire. He will do more and better for us than to accomplish all our wishes. And because we can trust His wisdom and love, we should not ask Him to concede to our will but should seek to enter into and accomplish His purpose. Our desires and interests should be lost in His will. These experiences that test faith are for our benefit. They reveal whether our faith is true and sincere, resting on the Word of God alone, or whether, depending on circumstances, it is uncertain and changeable. Faith is strengthened by exercise. We must let patience have its perfect work, remembering that there are precious promises in the Scriptures for those who wait upon the Lord.

Not all understand these principles. Many who seek the Lord's healing mercy think that they must have a direct and immediate answer to their prayers or their faith is defective. For this reason, those who are weakened by disease need to be counseled wisely, that they may act with discretion. They should not disregard their duty to the friends who may survive them, or neglect to employ nature's agencies for the restoration of health.

Often there is danger of error here. Believing that they will be healed in answer to prayer, some fear to do anything that might seem to indicate a lack of faith. But they should not neglect to set their affairs in order as they would desire to do if they expected to be removed by death. Nor should they fear to utter words of encouragement or counsel that at the parting hour they wish to speak to their loved ones.

Employ Remedial Agencies

Those who seek healing by prayer should not neglect to make use of the remedial agencies within their reach. It is not a denial of faith to use such remedies as God has provided to alleviate pain and to aid nature in her work of restoration. It is no denial of faith to cooperate with God and to place themselves in the condition most favorable to recovery. God has put it in our power to obtain a knowledge of the laws of life. This knowledge has been placed within our reach for use. We should employ every facility for the restoration of health, taking every advantage possible, working in harmony with natural laws. When we have prayed for the recovery of the sick, we can work with all the more energy, thanking God that we have the privilege of cooperating with Him, and asking His blessing on the means that He Himself has provided.

We have the sanction of the Word of God for the use of remedial agencies. Hezekiah, king of Israel, was sick, and a prophet of God brought him the message that he would die. He cried to the Lord, and the Lord heard His servant and sent him a message that fifteen years would be added to his life. One word from God would have healed Hezekiah instantly, but special directions were given, "'Let them take a lump of figs, and apply it as a poultice on the boil, and he shall recover.'" Isaiah 38:21.

On one occasion Christ used clay to anoint the eyes of a blind man and told him, "'Go, wash in the pool of Siloam'. . . . So he went and washed, and came back seeing." John 9:7. The cure could be wrought only by the power of the Great Healer, yet Christ made use of the simple agencies of nature. He did not give approval for drug medication, but He sanctioned the use of simple and natural remedies.

When we have prayed for the recovery of the sick, whatever the outcome, let us not lose faith in God. If we are called upon to meet bereavement, let us accept the bitter cup, remembering that a Father's hand holds it to our lips. But if health is restored, it should not be forgotten that the recipient of healing mercy is placed under renewed obligation to the Creator.

When the ten lepers were cleansed, only one returned to find Jesus and give Him glory. Let none of us be like the unthinking nine, whose hearts were untouched by the mercy of God. "Every good gift and every perfect gift is from above, and comes down from the Father of lights, with whom there is no variation or shadow of turning." James 1:17.

The Use
of Remedies

Disease never comes without a cause. The way is prepared and disease invited by disregard of the laws of health. Many suffer in consequence of the transgression of their parents. While they are not responsible for what their parents have done, nevertheless it is their duty to ascertain what are and what are not violations of the laws of health. They should avoid the wrong habits of their parents and, by correct living, place themselves in better conditions.

The greater number, however, suffer because of their own wrong course of action. They disregard the principles of health by their habits of eating, drinking, dressing, and working. Their transgression of nature's laws produces the sure result. Unfortunately, when sickness comes upon them, many do not credit their suffering to the true cause. They murmur against God because of their afflictions. But God is not responsible for the suffering that follows disregard of natural law.

God has endowed us with a reservoir of strength and vitality. He has also formed us with organs suited to maintain the various functions of life, and He designs that these organs shall work together in harmony. If we carefully preserve our God-given strength and keep the delicate mechanism of the body in order, the result is health; but if we use our strength recklessly and wastefully, the nervous system borrows power for present use from its resources of strength, and when one organ is injured, all are affected. Nature bears much abuse without apparent resistance, but then she arouses and makes a determined effort to remove the effects of the ill-treatment she has suffered. Her effort to correct these conditions is often manifested in fever and various other forms of sickness.

Rational Remedies

When the abuse of health is carried so far that sickness results, the sufferer can often do for himself or herself what no one else can do. The first thing to do is to ascertain the true character of the sickness and then go to work intelligently to remove the cause. If the harmonious working of the system has become unbalanced by overwork, overeating, or other irregularities, do not endeavor to adjust the difficulties by adding a burden of poisonous medicines.

Intemperate eating is often the cause of sickness, and what nature most needs is to be relieved of the undue burden that has been placed upon her. In many cases of sickness, the very best remedy is for the patient to fast for a meal or two, that the overworked organs of digestion may have an opportunity to rest. A fruit diet for a few days has often brought great relief to brain workers. Many times a short period of entire abstinence from food, followed by simple, moderate eating, has led to recovery through nature's own recuperative effort. A temperate diet for a month or two would convince many sufferers that the path of self-denial is the path to health.

Rest As a Remedy

Some make themselves sick by overwork. For these, rest, freedom from care, and a spare diet are essential to restoration of health. To those who are brain weary and nervous because of continual work and close confinement, a visit to the country, where they can live a simple, care-free life, coming in close contact with the things of nature, will be most helpful. Taking walks through the fields and woods, picking flowers, listening to the songs of the birds will do far more than any other agency toward their recovery.

In health and in sickness, pure water is one of Heaven's choicest blessings. Its proper use promotes health. It is the beverage that God provided to quench the thirst of animals and humans. Drunk freely, it helps to supply the necessities of the system and assists nature to resist disease. The external application of water is one of the easiest and most satisfactory ways of regulating the circulation of the blood. A cold or cool bath is an excellent tonic. Warm baths open the pores and thus aid in the elimination of impurities. Both warm and neutral baths soothe the nerves and equalize the circulation. But many have never learned by experience the beneficial effects of the proper use of water. Water treatments are not appreciated as they should be, and to apply them skillfully requires work that many are unwilling to perform.

But none should feel excused for ignorance or indifference on this subject. There are many ways in which water can be applied to relieve pain and check disease. All should become intelligent in its use in simple home treatments. Mothers, especially, should know how to care for their families in both health and sickness.

The Benefits of Activity

Action is a law of our being. Every organ of the body has its appointed work, upon the performance of which its development and strength depend. The normal action of all the organs gives strength and vigor, while the tendency of disuse is toward decay and death. Bind up an arm, even for a few weeks, then free it from its bands, and you will see that it is weaker than the arm you have been using moderately during the same time. Inactivity produces the same effect on the whole muscular system.

Inactivity is a fruitful cause of disease. Exercise quickens and equalizes the circulation of the blood, but in idleness the blood does not circulate freely, and the changes in it, so necessary to life and health, do not take place. The skin, too, becomes inactive. Impurities are not expelled as they would be if the circulation had been quickened by vigorous exercise, the skin kept in a healthy condition, and the lungs supplied with plenty of pure, fresh air. This state of the system throws a double burden on the excretory organs, and disease is the result.

Invalids should not be encouraged in inactivity. When there has been serious overtaxation in any direction, entire rest for a time will sometimes ward off serious illness, but in the case of confirmed invalids it is seldom necessary to suspend all activity.

Those who have broken down from mental work should have rest from wearing thought, but they should not be led to believe that it is dangerous to use their mental powers at all. Many are inclined to regard their condition as worse than it really is. This state of mind is unfavorable to recovery and should not be encouraged.

Ministers, teachers, students, and other brain workers often suffer from illness as the result of severe mental taxation, unrelieved by physical exercise. What these persons need is a more active life. Strictly temperate habits, combined with proper exercise, would ensure both mental and physical vigor and would give power of endurance to all brain workers. Those who have overtaxed their physical powers should not be encouraged to forgo manual labor entirely. But work, to be of the greatest advantage, should be systematic and agreeable. Outdoor exercise is the best; it should be so planned as to strengthen by use the organs that have become weakened. And the heart should be in it. Manual labor should never degenerate into mere drudgery.

When invalids have nothing to occupy their time and attention, their thoughts become centered upon themselves, and they grow morbid and irritable. Many times they dwell upon their bad feelings until they think they are much worse off than they really are and wholly unable to do anything.

In all these cases well-directed physical exercise would prove an effective remedial agent. In some cases it is indispensable to the recovery of health. The will goes with the labor of the hands, and what these invalids need is to have the will aroused. When the will is dormant, the imagination becomes abnormal, and it is impossible to resist disease.

Inactivity is the greatest curse that could come upon most invalids. Light employment in useful work does not tax either mind or body but has a beneficial influence on both. It strengthens the muscles, improves the circulation, and gives invalids the satisfaction of knowing that they are not wholly useless in this busy world. They may be able to do but little at first, but they will soon find their strength increasing, and the amount of work done can be increased accordingly.

Exercise aids a person with indigestion by giving the digestive organs a healthy tone. To engage in severe study or violent physical exercise immediately after eating hinders the work of digestion, but a short walk after a meal, with the head erect and the shoulders back, is a great benefit.

Many people neglect physical exercise in spite of all that is said and written concerning its importance. Some grow obese because the system is clogged. Others become thin and feeble because their strength is exhausted in disposing of an excess of food. The liver is burdened in its effort to cleanse the blood of impurities, and illness is the result.

Those whose habits are sedentary should, when the weather permits, exercise in the open air every day, summer or winter. Walking is preferable to riding or driving, for it brings more of the muscles into exercise. The lungs are forced into healthy action, since it is impossible to walk briskly without inflating them.

Such exercise would in many cases do more than medicine to improve one's health. Physicians often advise their patients to take an ocean voyage, go to some mineral spring, or visit some place with a different climate, when in most cases if the sick would eat temperately and take cheerful, healthful exercise, they would recover health. Plus, they would save time and money.

C h a p t e r 18

Mind
Cure

The relation that exists between the mind and the body is very intimate. When either one is affected, the other sympathizes. The condition of the mind affects the health to a far greater degree than many realize. Many of the diseases from which people suffer are the result of mental depression. Grief, anxiety, discontent, remorse, guilt, distrust, all tend to break down the life forces and to invite decay and death.

Disease is sometimes produced, and is often greatly aggravated, by the imagination. Many are lifelong invalids who might be well if they only thought so. Many imagine that every slight exposure will cause illness, and the evil effect is produced because it is expected. Many die from disease the cause of which is wholly imaginary.

Courage, hope, faith, sympathy, love promote health and prolong life. A contented mind, a cheerful spirit, is health to the body and strength to the soul. "A merry [rejoicing] heart does good, like medicine." Proverbs 17:22.

In the treatment of the sick, the effect of mental influence should not be overlooked. Rightly used, this influence affords one of the most effective agencies for combating disease.

Control of Mind Over Mind

There is, however, a form of mind cure that is one of the most effective agencies for evil. Through this so-called science, one mind is brought under the control of another so that the individuality of the weaker is merged in that of the stronger mind. One person acts out the will of another. Thus it is claimed that the tenor of the thoughts may be changed, that health-giving impulses may be imparted, and patients may be enabled to resist and overcome disease.

This method of cure has been employed by persons who were ignorant of its real nature and tendency and who believed it to be a means of benefit to the sick. But this so-called science is based upon false principles. It is foreign to the nature and spirit of Christ. It does not lead people to Him who is life and salvation. It leads them to separate from the true Source of their strength.

It is not God's purpose that human beings should yield mind and will to the control of another, becoming passive instruments. They are not to merge their individuality in that of another human being. They are not to look to any human being as the source of healing. Their dependence must be in God. In the dignity of their God-given personhood they are to be controlled by God Himself, not by any human intelligence.

God desires to bring us into direct relation with Himself. In all His dealings with human beings, He recognizes the principle of personal responsibility. He seeks to encourage a sense of personal dependence and to impress the need of personal guidance. He desires to bring the human into association with the divine, that we may be transformed into the divine likeness. Satan works to thwart this purpose. He seeks to encourage dependence upon humans. When minds are turned away from God, the tempter can bring them under his rule. He can control humanity.

The theory of mind controlling mind was originated by Satan to introduce himself as the chief worker, to put human philosophy where divine philosophy should be. Of all the errors that are finding acceptance among professedly Christian people, none is a more dangerous deception than this, none more certain to separate souls from God. Innocent though it may appear, if exercised upon patients, it will tend to their destruction, not to their restoration. It opens a door through which Satan will enter to take possession both of the mind that is given up to be controlled by another and of the mind that controls.

Fearful is the power thus given to evil-minded men and women. What opportunities it affords to those who live by taking advantage of others' weaknesses or follies! How many, through control of minds feeble or diseased, will find a means of gratifying lustful passion or greed of gain!

There is something better for us to engage in than the control of humanity by humanity. Physicians should educate people to look from the human to the divine. Instead of teaching people to depend upon human beings for the cure of soul and body, they should direct the sick to the One who can save to the uttermost all who come to Him. He who made the human mind knows what the mind needs. God alone is the One who can heal. Those whose minds and bodies are diseased are to behold in Christ the Restorer. "'Because I live,'" He says, "'you will live also.'" John 14:19.

This is the life we are to present to the sick, telling them that if they have faith in Christ as the Restorer, if they cooperate with Him, obeying the laws of health and striving to perfect holiness in His fear, He will impart to them His life. When we present Christ to them in this way, we are imparting a power, a strength, that is of value, for it comes from above. This is the true science of healing for body and soul.

Sympathy

Great wisdom is needed in dealing with diseases caused through the mind. A sore, sick heart, a discouraged mind, needs mild treatment. Many times some continuing home trouble is, like a canker, eating to the very soul and weakening one's hold on life. Sometimes remorse for sin undermines the constitution and unbalances the mind. Tender sympathy can benefit this class of invalids. The physician should first gain their confidence and then point them to the Great Healer. If their faith can be directed to the True Physician, and they can have confidence that He has undertaken their case, this will bring relief to the mind and often give health to the body.

Sympathy and tact will often prove a greater benefit to the sick than will skillful treatment given in a cold, indifferent way. When a physician comes to the sickbed in a listless, careless manner, looks at the afflicted one with little concern, by word or action giving the impression that the case requires scant attention, and then leaves the patient to his or her own reflections, he has done positive harm. The doubt and discouragement produced by his indifference will often counteract the good effect of the remedies he may prescribe.

If physicians could put themselves in the place of the one whose spirit is humbled, whose will is weakened by suffering, and who longs for words of sympathy and assurance, they would be better prepared to be empathetic. When the love and sympathy that Christ manifested for the sick is combined with medical knowledge, the physician's very presence will be a blessing.

Frankness inspires a patient with confidence and thus proves an important aid to recovery. There are physicians who consider it wise policy to conceal from the patient the nature and cause of the disease from which he or she is suffering. Many, fearing to excite or discourage patients by stating the truth, will hold out false hopes of recovery and even allow them to go down to the grave without warning them of their danger. All this is unwise.

It may not always be safe or best to explain to patients the full extent of their danger. This might alarm them and retard or even prevent recovery. Nor can the whole truth always be told to those whose ailments are largely imaginary. Many of these persons are unreasonable and have not accustomed themselves to exercise self-control. They have peculiar fancies and imagine many things that are false in regard to themselves and to others. To them these things are real, and those who care for them need to manifest constant kindness and unwearied patience and tact. If these patients were told the truth in regard to themselves, some would be offended, others discouraged. Christ said to His disciples, "'I still have many things to say to you, but you cannot bear them now.'" John 16:12.

But though not all the truth may be spoken on every occasion, it is never necessary or justifiable to deceive. Never should the physician or nurse stoop to prevarication. Those who do this place themselves where God cannot co-operate with them, and in forfeiting the confidence of their patients, they are casting away one of the most effective human aids to their restoration.

The power of the will is not valued as it should be. The will, kept awake and rightly directed, will impart energy to the whole being and will be a wonderful aid in maintaining health. It is a power also in dealing with disease. Exercised in the right direction, it would control the imagination and be a potent means of resisting and overcoming disease of both mind and body. By exercising will power in placing themselves in right relation to life, patients can do much to cooperate with the physician's efforts for their recovery.

There are thousands who can recover health if they will. The Lord does not want them to be sick. He wants them to be well and happy, and they should make up their minds to be well. Often invalids can resist disease simply by refusing to yield to ailments and being inactive. Rising above their aches and pains, let them engage in useful employment suited to their strength. By such employment and the free use of air and sunlight, many an emaciated invalid might recover health and strength.

Bible Principles of Cure

For those who would regain or preserve health there is a lesson in the words of Scripture, "Do not be drunk with wine, in which is dissipation; but be filled with the Spirit." Ephesians 5:18. Not through the excitement or oblivion produced by unnatural or unhealthful stimulants, not through indulgence of the lower appetites or passions is to be found true healing or refreshment for body or soul. Among the sick are many who are without God and without hope. They suffer from ungratified desires, disordered passions, and a condemning conscience. They are losing their hold on this life, and they have no prospect for the life to come.

Care givers should not hope to benefit these patients by granting them frivolous, exciting indulgences. These have been the curse of their lives. The hungry, thirsting soul will continue to hunger and thirst so long as it seeks to find satisfaction here. Those who drink at the fountain of selfish pleasure are deceived. They mistake hilarity for strength, and when the excitement ceases, their inspiration ends and they are left to discontent and despondency.

Abiding peace, true rest of spirit, has but one Source. Christ spoke of this when He said, "'Come to Me, all you who labor and are heavy laden, and I will give you rest.'" Matthew 11:28. "'Peace I leave with you, My peace I give to you; not as the world gives do I give to you.'" John 14:27. This peace is not something that He gives apart from Himself. It is in Christ, and we can receive it only by receiving Him.

Christ is the wellspring of life. That which many need is to have a clearer knowledge of Him. Patiently and kindly, yet earnestly, they need to be taught how the whole being may be thrown open to the healing agencies of Heaven. When the sunlight of God's love illuminates the darkened chambers of the soul, restless fatigue and dissatisfaction will cease, and satisfying joys will give vigor to the mind and health and energy to the body.

We are in a world of suffering. Difficulty, trial, and sorrow await us all along the way to our heavenly home. But there are many who make life's burdens doubly heavy by continually anticipating trouble. If they meet with adversity or disappointment, they think that everything is going to ruin, that theirs is the hardest lot of all, that they are surely coming to want. Thus they bring wretchedness upon themselves and cast a shadow upon all around them. Life itself becomes a burden to them.

But it need not be thus. It will require a determined effort to change the current of their thought. But the change can be made. Their happiness, both for this life and for the life to come, depends upon fixing their minds on cheerful things. Encourage them to look away from the dark picture, which is imaginary, to the benefits that God has strewn in their pathway, and beyond these to the unseen and eternal.

For every trial, God has provided help. When Israel in the desert came to the bitter waters of Marah, Moses cried to the Lord. The Lord did not provide some new remedy; He called attention to something that was at hand. A shrub that He had created was to be cast into the fountain to make the water pure and sweet. When this was done, the people drank of the water and were refreshed. In every trial, if we seek Christ, He will give us help. Our eyes will be opened to discern the healing promises recorded in His Word. The Holy Spirit will teach us how to appropriate every blessing that will be an antidote to grief. For every bitter drink that is placed to our lips, we shall find a branch of healing.

We are not to let the future, with its hard problems, its unsatisfying prospects, make our hearts faint, our knees tremble, our hands hang down. " 'Let him take hold of My strength,' " says the Mighty One, " 'that he may make peace with Me; and he shall make peace with Me.' " Isaiah 27:5. Those who surrender their lives to the guidance and service of God will never be placed in a position for which He has not made provision. Whatever our situation, if we are doers of His word, we have a Guide to direct our way. Whatever our perplexity, we have a sure Counselor. Whatever our sorrow, bereavement, or loneliness, we have a sympathizing Friend.

If in our ignorance we make missteps, the Savior does not forsake us. We need never feel that we are alone. Angels are our companions. The Comforter that Christ promised to send in His name abides with us. In the way that leads to the City of God, there are no difficulties that those who trust in Him may not overcome. There are no dangers that they may not escape. There is not a sorrow, not a grievance, not a human weakness, for which He has not provided a remedy.

None need abandon themselves to discouragement and despair. Satan may come to you with the cruel suggestion, "Yours is a hopeless case. You are irredeemable." But there is hope for you in Christ. God does not tell us to overcome in our own strength. He asks us to come close to His side. Whatever may be the difficulties that weigh down soul and body, He waits to set us free.

He who took humanity upon Himself knows how to sympathize with the sufferings of humanity. Not only does Christ know every soul and the peculiar needs and trials of that soul, He knows all the circumstances that chafe and perplex the spirit. His hand is outstretched in pitying tenderness to every suffering mortal. Those who suffer most have most of His sympathy and pity. He is touched with the feeling of our infirmities, and He desires us not only to lay our perplexities and troubles at His feet but to leave them there.

It is not wise to look to ourselves and study our emotions. Should we do this, the enemy will present difficulties and temptations that weaken faith and destroy courage. If we study closely our emotions and give way to our feelings, we shall entertain doubt and entangle ourselves in perplexity. We are to look away from self to Jesus.

When temptations assail you, when care, perplexity, and darkness seem to surround your soul, look to the place where you last saw the light. Rest in Christ's love and under His protecting care. When sin struggles for mastery of your heart, when guilt oppresses the soul and burdens the conscience, when unbelief clouds the mind, remember that Christ's grace is sufficient to subdue sin and banish the darkness. Entering into communion with the Savior, you enter the region of peace.

The Healing Promises

"The Lord redeems the soul of His servants,
And none of those who trust in Him shall be condemned."
Psalm 34:22.

"In the fear of the Lord there is strong confidence,
And His children will have a place of refuge."
Proverbs 14:26.

"Zion said, 'The Lord has forsaken me,
And my Lord has forgotten me.'
'Can a woman forget her nursing child,
And not have compassion on the son of her womb?
Surely they may forget,
Yet I will not forget you.
See, I have inscribed you on the palms of My hands.'"
Isaiah 49:14-16.

" ' "Fear not; for I am with you;
Be not dismayed, for I am your God.
I will strengthen you, Yes, I will help you,
I will uphold you with My righteous right hand." ' "

Isaiah 41:10.

Nothing tends more to promote health of body and of soul than does a spirit of gratitude and praise. It is a positive duty to resist melancholy, discontented thoughts and feelings—as much a duty as it is to pray. If we are heaven-bound, how can we go as a band of mourners, groaning and complaining all along the way to our Father's house?

Those professed Christians who constantly complain, and who seem to think that cheerfulness and happiness are a sin, do not have genuine religion. Those who take mournful pleasure in all that is melancholy in the natural world, who choose to look upon dead leaves rather than gather beautiful living flowers, who see no beauty in grand mountain heights and in valleys clothed with living green, who close their senses to the joyful voice that speaks to them in nature, and which is sweet and musical to the listening ear—these are not in Christ. They are gathering to themselves gloom and darkness when they might have brightness, even the Sun of Righteousness arising in their hearts with healing in His beams.

Often your mind may be clouded because of pain. Then do not try to think. You know that Jesus loves you. He understands your weakness. You may do His will by simply resting in His arms.

It is a law of nature that our thoughts and feelings are encouraged and strengthened as we give them utterance. While words express thoughts, it is also true that thoughts follow words. If we would give more expression to our faith, rejoice more in the blessings that we know we have—the great mercy and love of God—we would have more faith and greater joy. No tongue can express, no finite mind can conceive the blessing that results from appreciating the goodness and love of God. Even on earth we may have joy as a wellspring, never failing, because fed by the streams that flow from the throne of God.

Then let us educate our hearts and lips to speak the praise of God for His matchless love. Let us educate our souls to be hopeful and to abide in the light shining from the cross of Calvary. Never should we forget that we are children of the heavenly King, sons and daughters of the Lord of hosts. It is our privilege to maintain a calm repose in God.

"Let the peace of God rule in your hearts, . . . and be thankful." Colossians 3:15. Forgetting our own difficulties and troubles, let us praise God for an opportunity to live for the glory of His name. Let the fresh blessings of each new day awaken praise in our hearts for these tokens of His loving care. When you open your eyes in the morning, thank God that He has kept you through the night. Thank Him for His peace in your heart.

Morning, noon, and night, let gratitude as a sweet perfume ascend to heaven.

When someone asks how you are feeling, do not try to think of something mournful to tell in order to gain sympathy. Do not talk of your lack of faith and your sorrows and sufferings. The tempter delights to hear such words. When talking on gloomy subjects, you are glorifying him. We are not to dwell on the great power of Satan to overcome us. Often we give ourselves into his hands by talking of his power. Let us talk instead of the great power of God to bind up all our interests with His own. Tell of the matchless power of Christ, and speak of His glory.

All heaven is interested in our salvation. The angels of God, thousands upon thousands, and ten thousand times ten thousand, are commissioned to minister to those who shall be heirs of salvation. They guard us against evil and press back the powers of darkness that are seeking our destruction. Have we not reason to be thankful every moment, thankful even when apparent difficulties stand in our pathway?

Sing Praises

Let praise and thanksgiving be expressed in song. When tempted, instead of giving utterance to our feelings, let us by faith lift up a song of thanksgiving to God.

We praise Thee, O God, for the Son of Thy love—
For Jesus who died and is now gone above.

We praise Thee, O God, for Thy Spirit of light,
Who has shown us our Savior, and scattered our night.

All glory and praise to the Lamb that was slain,
Who has borne all our sins, and has cleansed every stain.

All glory and praise to the God of all grace,
Who has bought us, and sought us, and guided our ways.

Revive us again; fill each heart with Thy love;
May each soul be rekindled with fire from above.

CHORUS:
Hallelujah! Thine the glory, Hallelujah! amen;
Hallelujah! Thine the glory, Revive us again.

Song is a weapon that we can always use against discouragement. As we thus open the heart to the sunlight of the Savior's presence, we shall have health and His blessing.

"Give thanks to the Lord, for He is good!
For His mercy endures forever.
Let the redeemed of the Lord say so,
Whom He has redeemed from the hand of the enemy."

"Sing to Him, sing psalms to Him;
Talk of all His wondrous works!
Glory in His holy name;
Let the hearts of those rejoice who seek the Lord!"

"For He satisfies the longing soul,
And fills the hungry soul with goodness.
Those who sat in darkness and in the shadow of death,
Bound in affliction and irons— . . .
They cried out to the Lord in their trouble,
And He saved them out of their distresses.
He brought them out of darkness and the shadow of death,
And broke their chains in pieces.
Oh, that men would give thanks to the Lord for His goodness,
And for His wonderful works to the children of men!"

"Why are you cast down, O my soul?
And why are you disquieted within me?
Hope in God;
For I shall yet praise Him,
The help of my countenance and my God."
        Psalms 107:1, 2; 105:2, 3; 107:9-15; 42:11.

"In everything give thanks; for this is the will of God in Christ Jesus for you." 1 Thessalonians 5:18. This command is an assurance that even the things that appear to be against us will work for our good. God would not bid us be thankful for that which would do us harm.

"The Lord is my light and my salvation;
Whom shall I fear?
The Lord is the strength of my life;
Of whom shall I be afraid? . . .
For in the time of trouble He shall hide me in His pavilion;
In the secret place of His tabernacle He shall hide me; . . .
I will offer sacrifices of joy in His tabernacle;
I will sing, yes, I will sing praises to the Lord."

"I waited patiently for the Lord;
And He inclined to me, and heard my cry.
He also brought me up out of a horrible pit,
Out of the miry clay,
And set my feet upon a rock,
And established my steps.
He has put a new song in my mouth—
Praise to our God."

"The Lord is my strength and my shield;
My heart trusted in Him, and I am helped;
Therefore my heart greatly rejoices,
And with my song I will praise Him."
                    Psalms 27:1, 5, 6; 40:1-3; 28:7.

One of the surest hindrances to the recovery of the sick is the centering of attention upon themselves. Many invalids feel that everyone should give them sympathy and help, when what they need is to have their attention turned away from themselves, to think of and care for others.

Often prayer is requested for the afflicted, the sorrowful, the discouraged; and this is right. We should pray that God will shed light into the darkened mind and comfort the sorrowful heart. But God answers prayer for those who place themselves in the channel of His blessings. So, besides offering prayer for these sorrowful ones, we should encourage them to try to help those more needy than themselves. The darkness will be dispelled from their own hearts as they try to help others. As we seek to comfort others with the comfort with which we are comforted, the blessing comes back to us.

The fifty-eighth chapter of Isaiah is a prescription for maladies of the body and of the soul. If we desire health and the true joy of life, we must put into practice the rules given in this scripture. Of the service acceptable to Him, and its blessings, the Lord says:

"'Is it not to share your bread with the hungry,
And that you bring to your house the poor who are cast out;
When you see the naked, that you cover him,
And not hide yourself from your own flesh?
Then your light shall break forth like the morning,
Your healing shall spring forth speedily,
And your righteousness shall go before you;
The glory of the Lord shall be your rear guard.
Then you shall call, and the Lord will answer;
You shall cry, and He will say, "Here I am."
If you take away the yoke from your midst,

The pointing of the finger, and speaking wickedness,
If you extend your soul to the hungry
And satisfy the afflicted soul;
Then your light shall dawn in the darkness,
And your darkness shall be as the noonday.
The Lord will guide you continually,
And satisfy your soul in drought,
And strengthen your bones;
You shall be like a watered garden,
And like a spring of water,
Whose waters do not fail.'"

Isaiah 58:7-11.

Good deeds are twice a blessing, benefiting both the giver and the receiver of the kindness. The consciousness of right-doing is one of the best medicines for diseased bodies and minds. When the mind is free and happy from a sense of duty well done and the satisfaction of giving happiness to others, the cheering, uplifting influence brings new life to the whole being.

If you are an invalid, instead of constantly wanting sympathy, seek to impart it. Let the burden of your own weakness and sorrow and pain be cast upon the compassionate Savior. Open your heart to His love, and let it flow out to others. Remember that all have trials hard to bear, temptations hard to resist, and you may do something to lighten these burdens. Express gratitude for the blessings you have; show appreciation for the attentions you receive. Keep the heart full of the precious promises of God, that you may bring forth from this treasure words that will be a comfort and strength to others. This will surround you with an atmosphere that will be helpful and uplifting. Let it be your aim to bless those around you, and you will find ways of being helpful, both to the members of your own family and to others.

If those who are suffering from ill health would forget self in their interest for others, if they would fulfill the Lord's command to minister to those more needy than themselves, they would realize the truthfulness of the prophetic promise, "Then your light shall break forth like the morning, and your healing shall spring forth speedily."

Marah and Elim

Today 'tis Elim with its palms and wells,
And happy shade for desert weariness;
'Twas Marah yesterday, all rock and sand,
Unshaded solitude and dreariness.
Yet the same desert holds them both, the same
Hot breezes wander o'er the lonely ground;
The same low stretch of valley shelters both,

And the same mountains compass them around.
So it is here with us on earth, and so
I do remember it has ever been;
The bitter and the sweet, the grief and joy,
Lie near together, but a day between.

Sometimes God turns our bitter into sweet,
Sometimes He gives us pleasant watersprings;
Sometimes He shades us with His pillar cloud,
And sometimes to a blessed palm shade brings.

What matters it? The time will not be long;
Marah and Elim will alike be passed;
Our desert wells and palms will soon be done,
We reach the "City of our God" at last.
O happy land! beyond these lonely hills,
Where gush in joy the everlasting springs;
O holy Paradise! above these heavens,
Where we shall end our desert wanderings.
                    —Horatius Bonar.

Blessed Assurance

Blessed assurance, Jesus is mine!
Oh, what a foretaste of glory divine!
Heir of salvation, purchase of God,
Born of His Spirit, washed in His blood.

CHORUS:
This is my story, this is my song,
Praising my Savior all the day long;
This is my story, this is my song,
Praising my Savior all the day long.

Perfect submission, perfect delight,
Visions of rapture now burst on my sight.
Angels descending bring from above
Echoes of mercy, whispers of love.

Perfect submission, all is at rest,
I in my Savior am happy and blest,
Watching and waiting, looking above,
Filled with His goodness, lost in His love.
                    —Fanny J. Crosby.

$\mathcal{C}$ *h a p t e r* 19

In Contact
With Nature

The Creator chose for our first parents the surroundings best adapted for their health and happiness. He did not place them in a palace or surround them with the artificial adornments and luxuries that so many today are struggling to obtain. He placed them in close touch with nature and in close communion with the holy ones of heaven.

In the garden that God prepared as a home for His children, graceful shrubs and delicate flowers greeted the eye at every turn. There were trees of every variety, many of them bearing fragrant and delicious fruit. On their branches the birds caroled their songs of praise. Under their shadow the creatures of the earth sported together without a fear.

Adam and Eve, in their untainted purity, delighted in the sights and sounds of Eden. God appointed them their work in the garden, "to tend and keep it." Genesis 2:15. Each day's efforts brought them health and gladness, and the happy pair greeted with joy the visits of their Creator, as in the cool of the day He walked and talked with them. Daily God taught them His lessons.

The plan of life that God appointed for our first parents has lessons for us. Although sin has cast its shadow over the earth, God wants His children to find delight in the works of His hands. The more closely His plan of life is followed, the more wonderfully will He work to restore suffering humanity. The sick need to be brought into close touch with nature. An outdoor life amid natural surroundings would work wonders for many a helpless and almost hopeless invalid.

The noise and excitement and confusion of the cities, their strained and artificial life, are most wearisome and exhausting to the sick. The air, fouled by smoke, dust, poisonous gases, and germs of disease, is a peril to life. The sick, for the most part shut within four walls, come almost to feel as if they were prisoners in their rooms. They look out on houses and pavements and hurrying crowds, with perhaps not even a glimpse of blue sky or sunshine, of grass or flower or tree. Shut up in this way, they brood over their suffering and sorrow and become a prey to their own sad thoughts.

And for those who are weak in moral power, the cities abound in dangers. In them, patients who have unnatural appetites to overcome are continually exposed to temptation. They need to be placed amid new surroundings where the current of their thoughts will be changed. They need to be placed under influences entirely different from those that have wrecked their lives. For a time remove them into a purer atmosphere, away from those influences that lead away from God.

Institutions for the care of the sick would be far more successful if they could be established away from the cities. And so far as possible, all who are seeking to recover health should place themselves amid country surroundings where they can have the benefit of outdoor life. Nature is God's physician. The pure air, the bright sunshine, the flowers and trees, the orchards and vineyards, and outdoor exercise amid these surroundings are health-giving, life-giving.

Benefits of the Outdoor Life

Physicians and nurses should encourage their patients to be much in the open air. Outdoor life is the only remedy that many invalids need. It has a wonderful power to heal diseases caused by the excitements and excesses of fashionable life, a life that weakens and destroys the powers of body, mind, and soul.

To invalids weary of city life, with its glare of bright lights and noise of the streets, how soothing and healing are the quiet and freedom of the country! How eagerly do they turn to the scenes of nature! How glad they would be to sit in the open air, rejoice in the sunshine, and breathe the fragrance of tree and flower! There are life-giving properties in the balsam of the pine and in the fragrance of the cedar and fir. Other trees also have properties that are health restoring.

To the chronic invalid, nothing so tends to restore health and happiness as living amid attractive country surroundings. Here the most helpless can sit or lie in the sunshine or in the shade of the trees. They have only to lift their eyes to see beautiful foliage. A sweet sense of restfulness and refreshing comes over them as they listen to the murmuring of the breezes. The drooping spirits revive. The waning strength is recruited. Unconsciously the mind becomes peaceful, the fevered pulse more calm and regular. As the sick grow stronger, they will venture to take a few steps to gather some of the colorful flowers, precious messengers of God's love to His afflicted family here below.

Plans should be made to keep patients out of doors. For those who are able to work, let some pleasant, easy employment be provided. Show them how agreeable and helpful this outdoor work is. Encourage them to breathe the fresh air. Teach them to breathe deeply and to exercise the abdominal muscles in breathing and speaking. This is an education that will be invaluable to them.

Exercise in the open air should be prescribed as a life-giving necessity. And for such exercise there is nothing better than the cultivation of the soil. Let patients have flower beds to care for or work to do in the orchard or vegetable garden. As they are encouraged to leave their rooms and spend time in the open air, cultivating flowers or doing some other light, pleasant work, their attention will be diverted from themselves and their sufferings.

The more that patients can be kept out of doors, the less care they will require. The more cheerful their surroundings, the more hopeful they will be. Shut up in the house, be it ever-so-elegantly furnished, they will grow fretful and gloomy. Surround them with the beautiful things of nature. Place them where they can see flowers growing and the birds singing, and their hearts will break into song in harmony with the songs of the birds. Relief will come to body and mind. The intellect will be awakened, the imagination quickened, and the mind prepared to appreciate the beauty of God's Word.

Direct Minds to God

In nature something may always be found to divert the attention of the sick from themselves and direct their thoughts to God. Surrounded by His wonderful works, their minds are uplifted from the things that are seen to the things that are unseen. The beauty of nature leads them to think of the heavenly home, where there will be nothing to mar the loveliness, nothing to taint or destroy, nothing to cause disease or death.

Let physicians and nurses draw lessons from nature that teach about God. Let them point the patients to Him whose hand has made the lofty trees, the grass, and the flowers. Encourage them to see in every bud and flower an expression of God's love for His children. He who cares for the birds and the flowers will care for the beings formed in His own image.

Out of doors, amid the things that God has made, breathing fresh, health-giving air, the sick can best be told of the new life in Christ. Here God's Word can be read. Here the light of Christ's righteousness can shine into hearts darkened by sin.

Oh, could I find, from day to day,
A nearness to my God,
Then would my hours glide sweet away,
While leaning on His word.

Lord, I desire with Thee to live
Anew from day to day,
In joys the world can never give,
Nor ever take away.

Blest Jesus, come, and rule my heart,
And make me wholly Thine,
That I may nevermore depart,
Nor grieve Thy love divine.
                              —Benjamin Cleveland.

Men and women who need physical and spiritual healing are to be brought into contact with those whose words and acts will draw them to Christ. They are to be brought under the influence of the great Medical Missionary who can heal both soul and body. They are to hear the story of the Savior's love, of the pardon freely provided for all who come to Him confessing their sins.

Under such influences as these, many suffering ones will be guided into the way of life. Angels of heaven cooperate with human instrumentalities in bringing encouragement and hope, joy and peace, to the hearts of the sick and suffering. Under such conditions the sick are doubly blessed, and many find health. The feeble step recovers its elasticity. The eye regains its brightness. The hopeless become hopeful. The once despondent countenance wears an expression of joy. The complaining tones of the voice give place to tones of cheerfulness and content.

As physical health is regained, men and women are better able to exercise that faith in Christ which secures the health of the soul. In the consciousness of sins forgiven there is inexpressible peace and joy and rest. The clouded hope of the Christian is brightened. The words express the belief, "God is our refuge and strength, a very present help in trouble." "Yea, though I walk through the valley of the shadow of death, I will fear no evil; for You are with me; Your rod and Your staff, they comfort me." "He gives power to the weak, and to those who have no might He increases strength." Psalm 46:1; 23:4; Isaiah 40:29.

My faith looks up to Thee,
Thou Lamb of Calvary,
Savior divine;

Now hear me while I pray,
Take all my guilt away,
Oh, let me from this day
Be wholly Thine.

May Thy rich grace impart
Strength to my fainting heart,
My zeal inspire;
As Thou hast died for me,
Oh, may my love to Thee
Pure, warm, and changeless be,
A living fire.

While life's dark maze I tread,
And griefs around me spread,
Be Thou my Guide;
Bid darkness turn to day,
Wipe sorrow's tears away,
Nor let me ever stray
From Thee aside.

                              —Ray Palmer.

Health Principles

General
Hygiene

The knowledge that the human body is to be a temple for God, a dwelling through which to reveal His glory, should be the highest incentive for us to care for and develop our physical powers. Fearfully and wonderfully has the Creator formed and fashioned the human frame, and He tells us to make it our study, understand its needs, and act our part in preserving it from harm and defilement.

The Circulation of the Blood

In order to have good health, we must have good blood, for the blood is the current of life. It repairs waste and nourishes the body. When supplied with the proper food elements, and cleansed and vitalized by contact with pure air, it carries life and vigor to every part of the system. The better the circulation, the better will this work be accomplished.

At every pulsation of the heart the blood should make its way quickly and easily to all parts of the body. Its circulation should not be hindered by tight clothing or by insufficient clothing of the extremities. Whatever hinders the circulation forces the blood back to the vital organs, producing congestion. Headache, cough, palpitation of the heart, or indigestion is often the result.

Respiration

In order to have good blood, we must breathe well. Full, deep inspirations of pure air, which fill the lungs with oxygen, purify the blood. They impart to it a bright color and send it, a life-giving current, to every part of the body. Good respiration soothes the nerves, stimulates the appetite, and aids digestion. And it induces sound, refreshing sleep.

The lungs should be allowed the greatest freedom possible. Their capacity is developed by free action; it diminishes if they are cramped and compressed. Ill effects follow the practice so common, especially in sedentary pursuits, of stooping at one's work. In this position it is impossible to breathe deeply. Superficial breathing soon becomes a habit, and the lungs lose their power to expand.

A similar effect is produced by tight clothing around the waist. Sufficient room is not given to the lower part of the chest. The abdominal muscles, which were designed to aid in breathing, do not have full play, hence the lungs do not take in a sufficient supply of oxygen. The blood moves sluggishly. The waste, poisonous matter, which should be thrown off in the exhalations from the lungs, is retained, and the blood becomes impure.

Not only the lungs, but the stomach, liver, and brain are affected. The skin becomes sallow. Digestion is retarded. The heart is depressed. The brain is clouded. The thoughts are confused. Gloom settles over the spirits. The whole system becomes depressed and inactive, and peculiarly susceptible to disease.

The lungs are constantly throwing off impurities, and they need to be constantly supplied with fresh air. Impure air does not afford the necessary supply of oxygen, and the blood passes to the brain and other organs without being vitalized. Hence the necessity of thorough ventilation. To live in close, ill-ventilated rooms, where the air is dead and unhealthful, weakens the entire system. It becomes peculiarly sensitive to the influence of cold, and a slight exposure induces disease. Close confinement indoors makes many men and women pale and feeble. They breathe the same air over and over until it becomes laden with poisonous matter thrown off through the lungs and pores, and impurities are thus conveyed back to the blood.

Ventilation and Sunlight

In the construction of buildings, whether for public purposes or as homes, care should be taken to provide for good ventilation and plenty of sunlight. Churches and schoolrooms are often faulty in this respect. Neglect of proper ventilation is responsible for much of the drowsiness and dullness that destroy the effect of many a sermon and make the teacher's work toilsome and ineffective.

So far as possible, all buildings intended for human habitation should be placed on high, well-drained ground. This will ensure a dry site and prevent the danger of disease from dampness and a foggy, unwholesome atmosphere. This matter is often too lightly regarded. Continuous ill-health, serious diseases, and many deaths result from the dampness and malaria of low-lying, ill-drained situations.

When constructing homes it is especially important to secure thorough ventilation and plenty of sunlight. Make provision for a current of air and an abundance of light in every room in the house. Sleeping rooms should be so arranged as to have a free circulation of air day and night. No room is suitable as a bedroom unless it can be thrown open daily to fresh air and sunshine. In most countries bedrooms need to be supplied with conveniences for heating, that they may be thoroughly warmed and dried in cold or wet weather.

The guest room should have equal care with the rooms intended for constant use. Like the other bedrooms, it should have air and sunshine and should be provided with some means of heating to dry out the dampness that always accumulates in a room not in constant use. Whoever sleeps in a sunless room, or occupies a bed that has not been thoroughly dried and aired, does so at the risk of health, and often of life.

In building, many make careful provision for their plants and flowers. The greenhouse or window devoted to their use is warm and sunny, for without warmth, air, and sunshine, plants will not live and flourish. If these conditions are necessary to the life of plants, how much more necessary are they for our own health and that of our families and guests!

If we want our homes to be the abiding place of health and happiness, we must place them above the tainted vapors and fog of the lowlands, and give free entrance to Heaven's life-giving agencies. Dispense with heavy curtains, open the windows and blinds, allow no vines, however beautiful, to shade the windows, and permit no trees to stand so near the house as to shut out the sunshine. Sunlight may fade the draperies and carpets and tarnish the picture frames, but it will bring a healthy glow to the cheeks of the children. Those who have senior citizens to provide for should remember that these especially need warm, comfortable rooms. Vigor declines as years advance, leaving less vitality with which to resist unhealthful influences, hence the greater necessity for the elderly to have plenty of sunlight and fresh, pure air.

Scrupulous cleanliness is essential to both physical and mental health. Impurities are constantly thrown off from the body through the skin. Its millions of pores are quickly clogged unless kept clean by frequent bathing, and the impurities that should pass off through the skin become an additional burden to the other organs of elimination.

Most persons would be benefited by a cool or tepid bath every day, morning or evening. Instead of increasing the liability to take cold, a bath, properly taken, fortifies against cold, because it improves the circulation; the blood is brought to the surface, and a more easy and regular flow is obtained. The mind and the body are alike invigorated. The muscles become more flexible, the intellect is sharpened. The bath is a soother of the nerves and promotes digestion. It helps the bowels, the stomach, and the liver, giving health and energy to each.

It is important also that the clothing be kept clean. Garments absorb the waste matter that passes off through the pores. If they are not frequently changed and washed, the impurities will be reabsorbed.

Every form of uncleanliness tends to disease. Death-producing germs abound in dark, neglected corners, in decaying refuse, in dampness and mold and must. No waste vegetables or piles of fallen leaves should be allowed to remain near the house to decay and poison the air. Nothing unclean or decaying should be tolerated within the home. In towns or cities regarded perfectly healthful, many an epidemic of fever has been traced to decaying matter about the dwelling of some careless householder.

Maximum cleanliness, plenty of sunlight, and careful attention to sanitation are essential to freedom from disease and to the cheerfulness and vigor of all who live in the home.

Hygiene Among the Israelites

In the teaching that God gave to Israel, preservation of health received careful attention. The people who had come from slavery, with the uncleanly and unhealthful habits that it engenders, were subjected to the strictest training in the wilderness before entering Canaan. Health principles were taught and sanitary laws enforced.

Prevention of Disease

Not only in their religious service but in all the affairs of daily life was observed the distinction between clean and unclean. All who came in contact with contagious or contaminating diseases were isolated from the encampment, and they were not permitted to return without thorough cleansing of both their person and clothing. In the case of one afflicted with a contaminating disease, the direction was given:

" ' "Every bed is unclean on which he . . . lies, and everything on which he sits shall be unclean. And whoever touches his bed shall wash his clothes and bathe in water, and be unclean until evening. He who sits on anything on which he sat . . . shall wash his clothes and bathe in water, and be unclean until evening. And he who touches the body of him . . . shall wash his clothes and bathe in water, and be unclean until evening. . . . Whoever touches anything that was under him shall be unclean until evening. He who carries any of those things shall wash his clothes and bathe in water, and be unclean until evening. And whomever [the one] touches, and has not rinsed his hands in water, he shall wash his clothes and bathe in water, and be unclean until evening. The vessel of earth that he . . . touches shall be broken, and every vessel of wood shall be rinsed in water.'" Leviticus 15:4-12.

The law concerning leprosy is also an illustration of the thoroughness with which these regulations were to be enforced:

"'All the days he [the leper] has the sore he shall be unclean. He is unclean, and he shall dwell alone; his dwelling shall be outside the camp. Also, if a garment has a leprous plague in it, whether it is a woolen garment or a linen garment, whether it is in the warp or woof of linen or wool, whether in leather or in anything made of leather, . . . the priest shall look at the plague. . . . If the plague has spread in the garment, either in the warp or in the woof, in the leather or in anything made of leather, the plague is an active leprosy. It is unclean. He shall therefore burn that garment in which is the plague, whether warp or woof, in wool or in linen, or anything of leather, for it is an active leprosy; it shall be burned in the fire.'" Leviticus 13:46-52.

So, too, a house that gave evidence of conditions that made it unsafe for habitation was destroyed. The priest was to "'break down the house, its stones, its timber, and all the plaster of the house, and he shall carry them outside the city to an unclean place. Moreover he who goes into the house at all while it is shut up shall be unclean until evening. And he who lies down in the house shall wash his clothes, and he who eats in the house shall wash his clothes.'" Leviticus 14:45-47.

Cleanliness

The necessity of personal cleanliness was taught in the most impressive manner. Before gathering at Mount Sinai to listen to the proclamation of the law by the voice of God, the people were required to wash both their persons and their clothing. This order was enforced on pain of death. No impurity was to be tolerated in the presence of God.

During the sojourn in the wilderness the Israelites were almost continually in the open air, where impurities would have less harmful effects than in close houses. But the strictest regard to cleanliness was required both within and without their tents. No refuse was allowed to remain within or about the encampment. The Lord said: "'The Lord your God walks in the midst of your camp, to deliver you and give your enemies over to you; therefore your camp shall be holy.'" Deuteronomy 23:14.

Diet

The distinction between clean and unclean was made in all matters of diet: "'"I am the Lord your God, who has separated you from the peoples. You shall therefore distinguish between clean beasts and unclean, between unclean birds and clean, and you shall not make yourselves abominable by beast or by bird, or by any kind of living thing . . . which I have separated from you as unclean."'" Leviticus 20:24, 25.

Many articles of food eaten freely by the heathen about them were forbidden to the Israelites. It was no arbitrary distinction that was made. The things prohibited were unwholesome. And the fact that they were pronounced unclean taught the lesson that the use of injurious foods is defiling. That which corrupts the body tends to corrupt the soul. It unfits the user for communion with God, unfits one for high and holy service.

In the Promised Land the discipline begun in the wilderness was continued under circumstances favorable to the formation of right habits. The people were not crowded together in cities, but each family had its own landed possession, ensuring the health-giving blessings of a natural, unperverted life.

Concerning the cruel, licentious practices of the Canaanites, who were dispossessed by Israel, the Lord said: "'"You shall not walk in the statutes of the nation which I am casting out before you; for they commit all these things, and therefore I abhor them."'" Verse 23. "'Nor shall you bring an abomination into your house, lest you be doomed to destruction like it.'" Deuteronomy 7:26.

In all the affairs of their daily life, the Israelites were taught the lesson set forth by the Holy Spirit: "Do you not know that you are the temple of God and that the Spirit of God dwells in you? If anyone defiles the temple of God, God will destroy him. For the temple of God is holy, which temple you are."1 Corinthians 3:16, 17.

Rejoicing

"A merry [rejoicing] heart does good, like medicine." Proverbs 17:22. Gratitude, rejoicing, benevolence, trust in God's love and care—these are health's greatest safeguards. To the Israelites they were to be the very keynote of life.

The journey made three times a year to the annual feasts at Jerusalem, the week's sojourn in booths during the Feast of Tabernacles, were opportunities for outdoor recreation and social life. These feasts were occasions of rejoicing, made sweeter and more tender by the hospitable welcome given to the stranger, the Levite, and the poor.

"Rejoice in every good thing which the Lord your God has given to you and your house, you and the Levite and the stranger who is among you." Deuteronomy 26:11.

So, in later years, when the law of God was read in Jerusalem to the captives who had returned from Babylon, and the people wept because of their transgressions, the gracious words were spoken: "'Do not mourn. . . . Go your way, eat the fat, drink the sweet, and send portions to those for whom nothing is prepared; for this day is holy to our Lord. Do not sorrow, for the joy of the Lord is your strength.'" Nehemiah 8:9, 10.

And it was published and proclaimed "in all their cities and in Jerusalem, saying, 'Go out to the mountain, and bring olive branches, branches of oil trees, myrtle branches, palm branches, and branches of leafy trees, to make booths, as it is written.' Then the people went out and brought them and made themselves booths, each on the roof of his house, or in their courtyards or the courts of the house of God, and in the open square of the Water Gate and in the open square of the Gate of Ephraim. So the whole congregation of those who had returned from the captivity made booths and sat under the booths. . . . And there was very great gladness." Verses 15-17.

God gave to Israel instruction in all the principles essential to physical as well as moral health, and it was concerning these principles no less than concerning those of the moral law that He commanded them:

"'These words which I command you today shall be in your heart; you shall teach them diligently to your children, and shall talk of them when you sit in your house, when you walk by the way, when you lie down, and when you rise up. You shall bind them as a sign on your hand, and they shall be as frontlets between your eyes. You shall write them on the doorposts of your house and on your gates.'" Deuteronomy 6:6-9.

"'When your son asks you in time to come, saying, "What is the meaning of the testimonies, the statutes, and the judgments which the Lord our God has commanded you?" then you shall say to your son: . . . "The Lord commanded us to observe all these statutes, to fear the Lord our God, for our good always, that He might preserve us alive, as it is this day."'" Verses 20-24.

If the Israelites had obeyed the instruction they received and profited by their advantages, they would have been the world's object lesson of health and prosperity. If they had lived according to God's plan, they would have been preserved from the diseases that afflicted other nations. They would have possessed physical strength and vigor of intellect above any other people and would have been the mightiest nation on earth. God said:

"'You shall be blessed above all peoples.'" Deuteronomy 7:14.

"'Today the Lord has proclaimed you to be His special people, just as He has promised you, that you should keep all His commandments, and that He will set you high above all nations which He has made, in praise, in name, and in honor, and that you may be a holy people to the Lord your God, just as He has spoken.'" Deuteronomy 26:18, 19.

"'And all these blessings shall come upon you and overtake you, because you obey the voice of the Lord your God: Blessed shall you be in the city, and blessed shall you be in the country. Blessed shall be the fruit of your body, the produce of your ground and the increase of your herds, the increase of your cattle and the offspring of your flocks. Blessed shall be your basket and your kneading bowl. Blessed shall you be when you come in, and blessed shall you be when you go out.'" Deuteronomy 28:2-6.

"'The Lord will command the blessing on you in your storehouses and in all to which you set your hand, and He will bless you in the land which the Lord your God is giving you. The Lord will establish you as a holy people to Himself, just as He has sworn to you, if you keep the commandments of the Lord your God and walk in His ways. Then all peoples of the earth shall see that you are called by the name of the Lord, and they shall be afraid of you. And the Lord will grant you plenty of goods, in the fruit of your body, in the increase of your livestock, and in the produce of your ground, in the land of which the Lord swore to your fathers to give you. The Lord will open to you His good treasure, the heavens, to give the rain to your land in its season, and to bless all the work of your hand. . . . And the Lord will make you the head and not the tail; you shall be above only, and not beneath, if you heed the commandments of the Lord your God, which I command you today, and are careful to observe them.'" Verses 8-13.

To Aaron the high priest and his sons the direction was given: "'"This is the way you shall bless the children of Israel. Say to them:

'The Lord bless you and keep you;
The Lord make His face shine upon you,
And be gracious to you;
The Lord lift up His countenance upon you,
And give you peace.'"
So they shall put My name on the children of Israel;
And I will bless them.'"

> Numbers 6:23-27.

"'As your days, so shall your strength be.
There is no one like the God of Jeshurun,
Who rides the heavens to help you,
And in His excellency on the clouds.
The eternal God is your refuge,
And underneath are the everlasting arms. . . .
Israel shall dwell in safety,
The fountain of Jacob alone,
In a land of grain and new wine;
His heavens shall also drop dew.
Happy are you, O Israel!
Who is like you, a people saved by the Lord,
The shield of your help
And the sword of your majesty!'"

> Deuteronomy 33:25-29.

The Israelites failed to fulfill God's purpose and thus failed to receive the blessings that might have been theirs. But in Joseph and Daniel, in Moses and Elisha and many others, we have noble examples of the results of the true plan of living. The same faithfulness today will produce like results. To us it is written:

"You are a chosen generation, a royal priesthood, a holy nation, His own special people, that you may proclaim the praises of Him who called you out of darkness into His marvelous light." 1 Peter 2:9.

"Blessed are those who trust in the Lord,
whose trust is the Lord."
They shall "flourish like the palm tree,
and grow like a cedar in Lebanon.
They are planted in the house of the Lord;
they flourish in the courts of our God.
In old age they still produce fruit;
they are always green and full of sap."

"Let your heart keep my commands;
For length of days and long life
And peace they will add to you. . . .
Then you will walk safely in your way,
And your foot will not stumble.
When you lie down, you will not be afraid;
Yes, you will lie down and your sleep will be sweet.
Do not be afraid of sudden terror,
Nor of trouble from the wicked when it comes;
For the Lord will be your confidence,
And will keep your foot from being caught."
Jeremiah 17:7, Psalm 92:12-14, NRSV;
Proverbs 3:1, 2, 23-26.

C h a p t e r   22

Dress

The Bible teaches modesty in dress. "In like manner also, that the women adorn themselves in modest apparel." 1 Timothy 2:9. This forbids display in dress. Any device designed to attract attention to the wearer or to excite admiration (e.g., gaudy colors, profuse ornamentation) is excluded from the modest apparel that God's Word enjoins.

Our dress is to be inexpensive—not with "gold or pearls or costly clothing." Verse 9.

Money is a trust from God. It is not ours to expend for the gratification of pride or ambition. In the hands of God's children it is food for the hungry and clothing for the naked. It is a defense to the oppressed, a means of health to the sick, a means of preaching the gospel to the poor. Happiness could be brought to many hearts if only the money that is now spent for show were used wisely. Consider the life of Christ. Study His character and be partakers with Him in His self-denial.

In the professed Christian world enough is spent for jewelry and needlessly expensive dress to feed all the hungry and to clothe the naked. Fashion and display absorb the means that might comfort the poor and suffering. They rob the world of the gospel of the Savior's love. Missions languish. Multitudes perish for want of Christian teaching. Beside our own doors and in foreign lands many are untaught and unsaved.

Inasmuch as God has overspread the earth with His bounties, filled its storehouses with the comforts of life, and freely given us a saving knowledge of His truth, what excuse can we offer for not meeting the needs of the widow and fatherless, the sick and suffering, the untaught and unsaved? In the day of God, when brought face to face with Him who gave His life for these needy ones, what excuse will we offer for spending time and money on indulgences that God has forbidden? Will not Christ say to us, "'I was hungry and you gave Me no food; I was thirsty and you gave Me no drink; . . . naked and you did not clothe Me, sick and in prison and you did not visit Me'"? Matthew 25:42, 43.

But our clothing, while modest and simple, should be of good quality, of becoming colors, and suited for service. It should be chosen for durability rather than display. It should provide warmth and proper protection. The wise woman described in the Proverbs "is not afraid of the snow for her household: for all her household are clothed with double garments." Proverbs 31:21, KJV margin.

Our clothing should be clean. Uncleanliness in dress is unhealthful, and thus defiling to both body and soul. "You are the temple of God. . . . If anyone defiles the temple of God, God will destroy him." 1 Corinthians 3:16, 17.

In all respects our apparel should be healthful. "Above all things," God desires us to "be in health"—health of body and of soul. And we are to be workers together with Him for the health of both soul and body. Both are promoted by healthful dress.

Our apparel should have the grace, the beauty, the appropriateness of natural simplicity. Christ has warned us against the pride of life, but not against its grace and natural beauty. He pointed to the flowers of the field, to the lily unfolding in its purity, and said, "'Even Solomon in all his glory was not arrayed like one of these.'" Matthew 6:29. Thus by the things of nature Christ illustrated the beauty that Heaven values—the modest grace, simplicity, purity, and appropriateness that would make our attire pleasing to Him.

The most beautiful clothing He urges us to wear on the soul. No outward adorning can compare in value or loveliness to that "gentle and quiet spirit" which in His sight is "very precious." 1 Peter 3:4.

To those who make the Savior's principles their guide, how precious are His words of promise: "'Why do you worry about clothing? . . . If God so clothes the grass of the field, which today is, and tomorrow is thrown into the oven, will He not much more clothe you? . . . Therefore do not worry, saying, . . . "What shall we wear?" . . . For your heavenly Father knows that you need all these things. But seek first the kingdom of God and His righteousness, and all these things shall be added to you.'" Matthew 6:28-33.

"You will keep him in perfect peace, whose mind is stayed on You, because he trusts in You." Isaiah 26:3.

Avoid Slavery to Fashion

What a contrast is this to the weariness, the unrest, the disease and wretchedness, that result from the rule of fashion! How contrary to the principles given in the Scriptures are many of the modes of dress that fashion prescribes! Think of the styles that have prevailed for the last few hundred years, or even for the last few decades. Many of them when not in style would be declared immodest. Many would be pronounced inappropriate for a refined, God-fearing, self-respecting woman.

Making changes in apparel merely for the sake of fashion is not sanctioned by the Word of God. Changing styles and adding elaborate, costly ornamentation not only squander the time and means of the rich, they lay waste the energies of mind and soul. They impose a heavy burden on the middle and poorer classes. Many who can hardly earn a livelihood, and who with simple patterns might make their own clothing, are compelled to resort to the dressmaker in order to be in fashion. Many a poor woman, for the sake of a stylish gown, has deprived herself of warm undergarments and paid the penalty with her life. Many another, coveting the display and elegance of the rich, has been enticed into paths of dishonesty and shame. Many a home is deprived of comforts, many a man is driven to embezzlement or bankruptcy, to satisfy the extravagant demands of his wife or children.

Many a woman forced to prepare for herself or her children the stylish costumes demanded by fashion is doomed to ceaseless drudgery. For the sake of fashion she sacrifices health and that calmness of spirit so essential to the right guidance of her children. Improvement of mind and heart is neglected. The soul is dwarfed.

The mother has no time to study the principles of physical development, that she may know how to care for the health of her children. She has no time for ministering to their mental or spiritual needs, no time to sympathize with them in their little disappointments and trials, or to share in their interests and pursuits.

Almost as soon as they come into the world, children are subjected to fashion's influence. They hear more of dress than of their Savior. They see their mothers consulting the fashion magazines more earnestly than the Bible. The display of dress is treated as of greater importance than the development of character. Parents and children are robbed of that which is best and sweetest and truest in life. For fashion's sake they are cheated out of a preparation for the life to come.

It was the adversary of all good who instigated the invention of the ever-changing fashions. He desires nothing so much as to bring grief and dishonor to God by making human beings miserable and ruining them. One of the means by which he most effectively accomplishes this is through the devices of fashion that weaken the body, enfeeble the mind, and belittle the soul.

Many women are subject to serious maladies, and their sufferings are greatly increased by their manner of dress. Instead of preserving their health for the trying emergencies that are sure to come, too often by their wrong habits they sacrifice not only health but life, and leave to their children a legacy of woe in poor health, perverted habits, and false ideas of life.

Any style of dress that cramps the lungs, making correct breathing difficult, should be avoided. It is essential to health that the chest have room to expand to its fullest extent in order that the lungs may be enabled to take full inspiration. When the lungs are restricted, the amount of oxygen received into them is lessened, and the waste, poisonous matter that should be thrown off through the lungs is retained.

Dress for Health and Beauty

One of the chief elements in physical beauty is symmetry, the harmonious proportion of parts. And the correct model for physical development is to be found not in the figures displayed by French designers but in the human form as developed according to the laws of God in nature. God is the author of all beauty, and only as we conform to His ideal shall we approach the standard of true beauty.

Another evil that custom fosters is the unequal distribution of the clothing, so that while some parts of the body have more than is required, others are insufficiently clad. The feet and limbs, being remote from the vital organs, should be especially guarded from cold by abundant clothing. It is impossible to have health when the extremities are habitually cold, for if there is too little blood in them there will be too much in other portions of the body. Perfect health requires perfect circulation, but this cannot be had while three or four times as much clothing is worn on the body where the vital organs are situated than on the feet and limbs.

A multitude of women are nervous and careworn because they deprive themselves of the pure air that would make pure blood and of the freedom of motion that would send the blood bounding through the veins, giving life, health, and energy. Many women have become confirmed invalids when they might have enjoyed health, and many have died of tuberculosis and other diseases when they might have lived their allotted term of life if they had dressed in accordance with health principles and exercised freely in the open air.

In order to secure the most healthful clothing, the needs of every part of the body must be carefully studied. The character of the climate, the surroundings, the condition of health, the age, and the occupation—all must be considered. Every article of dress should fit easily, obstructing neither the circulation of the blood nor free, full, natural breathing.

Women who are in failing health can do much for themselves by sensible dressing and by exercising. When suitably dressed for outdoor enjoyment, let them exercise in the open air, carefully at first but increasing the amount of exercise as they can endure it. By taking this course, many might regain health and live to take their share in the world's work.

Be Independent of Fashion

Instead of struggling to meet the demands of fashion, women should have the courage to dress healthfully and simply. Instead of sinking into a mere household drudge, the wife and mother should take time to read, keep herself well informed, be a companion to her husband, and keep in touch with the developing minds of her children. She should use wisely her opportunities to influence her dear ones for the higher life. She should take time to make the Savior a daily companion and familiar friend. She should take time for the study of His Word, take time to go with the children on nature walks, and learn of God through the beauty of His works.

Let her keep cheerful and buoyant. Make the evening a pleasant social season, a family reunion after the day's duties. Many a husband would thus be led to choose the society of his home before that of the clubhouse or bar. Many a son would be kept from spending time at the corner store or joining a street gang. Many a daughter would be saved from frivolous, misleading associations. The influence of the home would be to parents and children what God designed it to be—a lifelong blessing.

Chapter 23

Diet
and Health

Our bodies are built up from the food we eat. There is a constant breaking down of the tissues of the body. Every movement of every organ involves waste, and this waste is repaired from our food. Each organ of the body requires its share of nutrition. The brain must be supplied with its portion. The bones, muscles, and nerves demand theirs. It is a wonderful process that transforms the food into blood and uses this blood to build up the varied parts of the body. This process is going on continually, supplying with life and strength each nerve, muscle, and tissue.

Selection of Food

Those foods should be chosen that best supply the elements needed for building up the body. In making this choice, appetite is not a safe guide. Through wrong habits of eating, the appetite has become perverted. Often it demands food that impairs health and causes weakness instead of strength. We cannot be guided safely by the customs of society. The disease and suffering that everywhere prevail are largely due to popular errors in regard to diet.

In order to know what are the best foods, we must study God's original plan for our diet. He who created human beings and understands their needs appointed Adam his food. "' See,'" He said, "'I have given you every herb that yields seed . . . and every tree whose fruit yields seed; to you it shall be for food.'" Genesis 1:29. Upon leaving Eden to gain his livelihood by tilling the earth under the curse of sin, Adam received permission to eat also "'the herb of the field.'" Genesis 3:18.

Grains, fruits, nuts, and vegetables constitute the diet chosen for us by our Creator. These foods, prepared in as simple and natural a manner as possible, are the most healthful and nourishing. They impart a strength, a power of endurance, and a vigor of intellect that are not afforded by a more complex and stimulating diet.

But not all foods wholesome in themselves are equally suited to our needs under all circumstances. Care should be taken in the selection of food. Our diet should be suited to the season, to the climate in which we live, and to the occupation we follow. Some foods that are the best choice for use at one season or in one climate are not the best choice in another. Likewise, there are different foods best suited for persons in different occupations. Often food that can be used with benefit by those engaged in hard physical labor is unsuitable for persons of sedentary pursuits or intense mental application. God has given us an ample variety of healthful foods, and we should choose from it the things that experience and sound judgment prove to be best suited to our own individual necessities.

Nature's abundant supply of fruits, nuts, and grains is ample, and today, by the increased facilities for transportation, the products of all lands are more generally distributed to all. As a result, many articles of food that a few years ago were regarded as expensive luxuries are now within the reach of all. This is especially the case with dried and canned fruits.

Nuts and nut foods are coming largely into use to take the place of flesh meats. With nuts may be combined grains, fruits, and some roots to make foods that are healthful and nourishing. People who suffer ill effects from nuts may find complete relief by reducing the amount of nuts eaten. And keep in mind that some nuts are more wholesome than others. Almonds are preferable to peanuts, but peanuts in limited quantities, used in connection with grains, are nourishing and digestible.

When properly prepared, olives, like nuts, supply the place of butter and flesh meats. The oil, as eaten in the olive, is far preferable to animal oil or fat. It serves as a laxative. Its use will be found beneficial to people with tuberculosis, and it is healing to an inflamed, irritated stomach.

Persons who have accustomed themselves to a rich, highly stimulating diet have an unnatural taste, and they cannot at once relish food that is plain and simple. It will take time for the taste to become natural and for the stomach to recover from the abuse it has suffered. But those who persevere in the use of wholesome food will, after a time, find it palatable. Its delicate and delicious flavors will be appreciated, and it will be eaten with greater enjoyment than can be derived from unwholesome delicacies. And the stomach, in a healthy condition, neither fevered nor overtaxed, can readily perform its task.

In order to maintain health, a sufficient supply of good, nourishing food is needed. If we plan wisely, that which is most conducive to health can be secured in almost every land. The various preparations of rice, wheat, corn, and oats are sent abroad everywhere; also beans, peas, and lentils. These, with native or imported fruits and the variety of vegetables that grow in each locality, give an opportunity to select a dietary that is complete without the use of flesh meats.

Wherever fruit can be grown in abundance, a liberal supply should be prepared for winter by canning or drying. Small fruits, such as currants, gooseberries, strawberries, raspberries, and blackberries, can be grown to advantage in many places where they are but little used and their cultivation is neglected. For household canning, glass, rather than tin cans, should be used whenever possible. It is especially necessary that the fruit be in good condition. Use little sugar, and cook the fruit only long enough to ensure its preservation. Thus prepared, it is an excellent substitute for fresh fruit.

Wherever dried fruits, such as raisins, prunes, apples, pears, peaches, and apricots, are obtainable at moderate prices, it will be found that they can be used as staple articles of diet much more freely than is customary, with the best results to the health and vigor of all classes of workers.

There should not be a great variety at any one meal, for this encourages overeating and causes indigestion. It is not well to eat fruit and vegetables at the same meal. If the digestion is feeble, the use of both will often cause distress and inability to put forth mental effort. It is better to have the fruit at one meal and the vegetables at another. The meals should be varied. The same dishes, prepared in the same way, should not appear on the table meal after meal, day after day. Meals will be eaten with greater relish, and the system will be better nourished, when the food is varied.

Preparation of Food

It is wrong to eat merely for pleasure; nevertheless, one should not be indifferent to the quality of the food or how it is prepared. If the food eaten is not relished, the body will not be as well nourished. The food should be carefully chosen and prepared with intelligence and skill.

In breadmaking, superfine white flour is not the best. Its use is neither healthful nor economical. Fine-flour bread lacks nutritive elements to be found in bread made from the whole wheat. It is a frequent cause of constipation and other unhealthful conditions.

The use of soda or baking powder in breadmaking is harmful and unnecessary. Soda causes inflammation of the stomach and often poisons the entire system. Many housewives think that they cannot make good bread without soda, but this is an error. If they would take the trouble to learn better methods, their bread would be more wholesome, and, to a natural taste, it would be more palatable.

In the making of raised or yeast bread, use water instead of milk. Milk is an additional expense and makes the bread less wholesome. Milk bread does not keep sweet as long after baking as does that made with water, and it ferments more readily in the stomach. Bread should be light and sweet. Not the least taint of sourness should be tolerated. The loaves should be small and so thoroughly baked that, so far as possible, the yeast germs shall be destroyed. When hot or new, raised bread of any kind is difficult to digest. It should never appear on the table. This rule does not, however, apply to unleavened bread. Fresh rolls made of wheaten meal without yeast or leaven, and baked in a well-heated oven, are both wholesome and palatable.

Grains used as cereal should be well cooked. But soft or liquid foods are less wholesome than dry foods, which require thorough chewing. Zwieback, or twice-baked bread, is one of the most easily digested and most palatable of foods. Let ordinary raised bread be cut in slices and dried in a warm oven till the last trace of moisture disappears. Then let it be browned slightly all the way through. If kept dry, this bread will be good much longer than ordinary bread, and, if reheated before using, it will taste as fresh as when new.

Far too much sugar is ordinarily used in food. Cakes, sweet puddings, pastries, jellies, jams, are active causes of indigestion. Especially harmful are the custards and puddings in which milk, eggs, and sugar are the chief ingredients. The free use of milk and sugar taken together should be avoided.

If milk is used, it should be thoroughly sterilized. With this precaution, there is less danger of contracting disease from its use. Butter is less harmful when eaten on cold bread than when used in cooking, but as a rule it is better to dispense with it altogether. Cheese is still more objectionable; it is wholly unfit for food.*

Scanty, poorly cooked food depraves the blood by weakening the blood-making organs. It deranges the system and brings on disease, with its accompaniment of irritable nerves and bad tempers. The victims of poor cookery are numbered by thousands and tens of thousands. Over many graves might be written: "Died because of poor cooking," or "Died of an abused stomach."

It is a sacred duty for those who cook to learn how to prepare healthful food. Many souls are lost as the result of poor cookery. It takes thought and care to make good bread, but there is more religion in a loaf of good bread than many think. There are few really good cooks. Young women think that it is menial to cook and do other kinds of housework. For this reason many girls who marry and have the care of families have little idea of the duties devolving upon a wife and mother.

Cooking is no mean science, and it is one of the most essential in practical life. It is a science that both men and women might well learn,

---

*This is understood to mean ripened cheese.—Publisher.

and it should be taught in a way to benefit the poorer classes. To make food simple and nourishing and at the same time appetizing requires skill, but it can be done. Cooks should know how to prepare food not only in a simple and healthful manner, but so that it will be found more palatable as well as more wholesome because of its simplicity.

Every woman who is at the head of a family and yet does not understand the art of healthful cookery should determine to learn that which is so essential to the well-being of her household. In many places cooking schools afford opportunity for instruction in this line. She who has not the help of such facilities should put herself under the instruction of some good cook and persevere in her efforts for improvement until she masters the culinary art.

Regularity in eating is of vital importance. There should be a specified time for each meal. At this time let everyone eat what the system requires and then take nothing more until the next meal. There are many who eat when the system needs no food, at irregular intervals, and between meals, because they have not sufficient strength of will to resist inclination. When traveling, some are constantly nibbling if anything suitable to eat is within their reach. This is very injurious. If travelers would eat regularly of food that is simple and nutritious, they would not feel so tired nor suffer so much from sickness.

Another pernicious habit is that of eating just before bedtime. People may have eaten their regular meals, but because they feel faint, they eat more. By indulgence this wrong practice becomes a habit and often so firmly fixed that they think it is impossible to sleep without food. As a result of eating late suppers, the digestive process is continued through the sleeping hours. But though the stomach works constantly, its work is not properly accomplished. The sleep is often disturbed with unpleasant dreams, and in the morning the person awakes unrefreshed and with little relish for breakfast. When we lie down to rest, the stomach should be through with its work, so that it, as well as the other organs of the body, may enjoy rest. Late suppers are particularly harmful for persons of sedentary habits. With them the disturbance created is often the beginning of disease that ends in death.

In many cases the faintness that leads to a desire for food is felt because the digestive organs have been too severely taxed during the day. After disposing of one meal, the digestive organs need rest. At least five or six hours should elapse between meals, and most persons who give the plan a trial will find that two meals a day are better than three.

Wrong Conditions of Eating

When eaten, food should not be very hot or very cold. If food is cold, one's vitality is drawn upon in order to warm it before digestion can take place. Cold drinks are injurious for the same reason, while the free use of hot drinks is debilitating. In fact, the more liquid that is taken with meals, the more difficult it is for food to digest, for the liquid must be absorbed before digestion can begin. The irritation that calls for so much drink at mealtime will largely disappear if one uses little salt, avoids the use of pickles and spiced foods, and eats an abundance of fruit.

Food should be eaten slowly and thoroughly chewed. This is necessary in order that the saliva may mix properly with the food and the digestive fluids be called into action. Another serious evil is eating at improper times, as after violent or excessive exercise, when one is exhausted or overheated. Immediately after eating there is a strong demand upon the nervous energies, and when mind or body is heavily taxed just before or just after eating, digestion is hindered. When one is excited, anxious, or hurried, it is better not to eat until rest or relief is found.

The stomach is closely related to the brain. When the brain is constantly taxed and there is lack of physical exercise, even plain food should be eaten sparingly. At mealtime cast off care and anxious thought. Do not feel hurried. Eat slowly and be happy, with your heart filled with gratitude to God for all His blessings.

Many who discard flesh meats and other gross and injurious articles think that because their food is simple and wholesome they may indulge appetite without restraint. They eat to excess, sometimes to gluttony. This is an error. The digestive organs should not be burdened with a quantity or quality of food that will tax the system.

Custom has decreed that food shall be placed upon the table in courses. Not knowing what is coming next, people may eat an amount of food that perhaps is not best suited to them. When the last course is brought on, they often venture to overstep the bounds and take the tempting dessert, which, however, proves anything but good for them. If all the food intended for a meal is placed on the table at the beginning, one has opportunity to make the best choice.

Sometimes the result of overeating is felt at once. In other cases there is no sensation of pain, but the digestive organs become exhausted, and the foundation of physical strength is undermined.

The surplus food burdens the system and produces unhealthy, feverish conditions. It calls an undue amount of blood to the stomach, causing the limbs and extremities to chill quickly. It lays a heavy tax on the digestive organs, and when these organs have accomplished their task, there is a feeling of weakness or listlessness. Some who are continually overeating think this all-gone feeling is hunger, but it is caused by the overworked condition of the digestive organs. At times there is numbness of the brain, with disinclination to mental or physical effort.

These unpleasant symptoms are felt because nature has accomplished her work at an unnecessary outlay of strength and is thoroughly exhausted. The stomach is saying, "Give me rest." But with many the faintness is interpreted as a demand for more food, so, instead of giving the stomach rest, another burden is placed upon it. As a consequence the digestive organs are often worn out when they should be capable of doing good work.

We should not provide for the Sabbath a more liberal supply or a greater variety of food than for other days. Instead, the food should be more simple, and less should be eaten in order that the mind may be clear and vigorous to comprehend spiritual things. A clogged stomach means a clogged brain. The most precious words may be heard and not appreciated because the mind is confused by an improper diet. By overeating on the Sabbath, many do more than they think to unfit themselves for receiving the benefit of its sacred opportunities.

Cooking on the Sabbath should be avoided, but it is not necessary to eat cold food. In cold weather the food prepared the day before should be heated. And let the meals, however simple, be tasty and attractive. Especially in families where there are children, it is well, on the Sabbath, to provide something that will be regarded as a treat.

The Need for Reform

Where wrong habits of diet have been indulged, there should be no delay in reform. When chronic indigestion has resulted from abuse of the stomach, efforts should be made carefully to preserve one's remaining strength by removing every overtaxing burden. The stomach may never entirely recover health after long abuse, but a proper course of diet will save further debility, and many will recover more or less fully. It is not easy to prescribe rules that will meet every case, but with attention to right principles in eating, great reforms may be made, and the cook need not be continually trying to tempt the appetite.

Moderation in diet is rewarded with mental and moral vigor. It also aids in the control of the passions. Overeating is especially harmful to those who are sluggish in temperament. These should eat sparingly and take plenty of physical exercise. There are men and women of excellent natural ability who do not accomplish half what they might if they would exercise self-control in the denial of appetite.

Many writers and speakers fail here. After eating heartily, they give themselves to sedentary occupations, reading, studying, or writing, allowing no time for physical exercise. As a consequence, the free flow of thought and words is checked. They cannot write or speak with the force and intensity necessary in order to reach the heart. Their efforts are tame and fruitless.

Those upon whom rest important responsibilities, those, above all, who are guardians of spiritual interests, should be persons of keen feeling and quick perception. More than others, they need to be temperate in eating. Rich and luxurious food should have no place on their tables.

Every day people in positions of trust have decisions to make upon which depend results of great importance. Often they have to think rapidly, and they can do this successfully only if they practice strict temperance. The mind strengthens under the correct treatment of the physical and mental powers. If the strain is not too great, new vigor comes with every taxation. But often the work of those who have important plans to consider and important decisions to make is affected for evil by the results of improper diet. A disordered stomach produces a disordered, uncertain state of mind. Often it causes irritability, harshness, or injustice. Many a plan that would have been a blessing to the world has been discarded, many unjust, oppressive, even cruel measures have been enacted as the result of diseased conditions due to wrong habits of eating.

Let all whose work is sedentary or chiefly mental and who have sufficient moral courage and self-control try the following suggestion: At each meal take only two or three kinds of simple food, and eat no more than is required to satisfy hunger. Take active exercise every day, and see if you do not receive benefit.

Strong men who are engaged in active physical labor are not compelled to be as careful as to the quantity or quality of their food as are persons of sedentary habits, but even these would have better health if they would practice self-control in eating and drinking.

Some wish that an exact rule could be prescribed for their diet. They overeat, and then regret it, and so they keep thinking about what they eat and drink. This is not as it should be. One person cannot lay down an exact rule for another. Everyone should exercise reason and self-control, and should act from principle.

Our bodies are Christ's purchased possession, and we are not at liberty to do with them as we please. All who understand the laws of health should realize their obligation to obey these laws that God has established in their being. Obedience to the laws of health is to be made a matter of personal duty. We ourselves must suffer the results of violated law. We must individually answer to God for our habits and practices. Therefore the question with us is not, "What is the world's practice?" but, "How shall I as an individual treat the body that God has given me?"

Flesh
as Food

The diet appointed to human beings in the beginning did not include animal food. Not till after the Flood, when every green thing on the earth had been destroyed, did they receive permission to eat flesh.

In choosing their food in Eden, the Lord showed what was the best diet. In the choice made for Israel, He taught the same lesson. He brought the Israelites out of Egypt and undertook their training that they might be a people for His own possession. Through them He desired to bless and teach the world. He provided them with the food best adapted for this purpose, not flesh, but manna, "the bread of heaven." It was only because of their discontent and their murmuring for the fleshpots of Egypt that animal food was granted them, and this for only a short time. Its use brought disease and death to thousands. Yet the restriction to a nonflesh diet was never heartily accepted. It continued to be the cause of discontent and murmuring, open or secret, and it was not made permanent.

Upon their settlement in Canaan, the Israelites were permitted the use of animal food, but under careful restrictions that tended to lessen the evil results. The use of swine's flesh was prohibited as was also that of other animals, birds, and fish whose flesh was pronounced unclean. Clean meats were permitted, but eating of the fat and blood was strictly forbidden.

Only such animals could be used for food as were in good condition. No creature that was torn, that had died of itself, or from which the blood had not been carefully drained could be used as food. By departing from the plan divinely appointed for their diet, the Israelites suffered great loss.

They desired a flesh diet, and they reaped its results. They did not reach God's ideal of character or fulfill His purpose. The Lord "gave them their request, but sent leanness into their soul." Psalm 106:15. They valued the earthly above the spiritual, and they did not attain the sacred preeminence that was His purpose for them.

Reasons for Discarding Flesh Foods

Those who eat flesh are but eating grains and vegetables at second hand, for the animal receives from these things the nutrition that produces growth. The life that was in the grains and vegetables passes into the eater. We receive it by eating the flesh of the animal. How much better to get it directly, by eating the food that God provided for our use!

Flesh was never the best food, but its use is now doubly objectionable, since disease in animals is rapidly increasing. Those who use flesh foods little know what they are eating. Often if they could see the animals when living and know the quality of the meat they eat, they would turn from it with loathing. People are continually eating flesh that is filled with tuberculosis and cancerous germs. Tuberculosis, cancer, and other fatal diseases are thus communicated.

The tissues of the swine swarm with parasites. God said, "'The swine is unclean for you . . . ; you shall not eat their flesh or touch their dead carcasses.'" Deuteronomy 14:8. This command was given because swine's flesh is unfit for food. Swine are scavengers, and this is the only use they were intended to serve. Never, under any circumstances, was their flesh to be eaten by human beings. It is impossible for the flesh of any living creature to be wholesome when filth is its natural element and when it feeds on every detestable thing.

Often animals are taken to market and sold for food when they are so diseased that their owners fear to keep them longer. And some of the processes of fattening them for market produce disease. Shut away from the light and pure air, breathing the atmosphere of filthy stables, perhaps fattening on decaying food, the entire body soon becomes contaminated with foul matter.

To reach the market, animals are often transported long distances and subjected to great suffering. Taken from the green pastures, and traveling for weary miles over hot, dusty roads, they become feverish and exhausted. Often, crowded into filthy railroad cars or trucks and for many hours deprived of food and water, the poor creatures are driven to their death that human beings may feast on their carcasses.

In many places fish become so contaminated by the filth on which they feed as to be a cause of disease. This is especially the case where fish come in contact with the sewage of large cities. These fish may pass into distant waters and may be caught where the water is pure and fresh, but when used as food they bring disease and death on those who do not suspect the danger.

The effects of a flesh diet may not be immediately realized, but this is no evidence that it is not harmful. Few can be made to believe that it is the meat they have eaten that has poisoned their blood and caused them suffering. Many die of diseases wholly due to meat eating, while the real cause is not suspected by themselves or by others.

The moral evils of a flesh diet are not less marked than are the physical ills. Flesh food is injurious to health, and whatever affects the body has a corresponding effect on the mind and soul. Think of the cruelty to animals that meat eating involves. Think of its effect on those who inflict the cruelty and on those who behold it. How it destroys the tenderness with which we should regard these creatures of God!

The intelligence displayed by many dumb animals approaches so closely to human intelligence that it is a mystery. The animals see and hear and love and fear and suffer. They use their organs far more faithfully than many human beings use theirs. They manifest sympathy and tenderness toward their companions in suffering. Many animals show an affection for those who have charge of them, far superior to the affection shown by some of the human race. They form attachments for humans that are not broken without great suffering to them.

What person with a human heart, who has ever cared for domestic animals, could look into their eyes, so full of confidence and affection, and willingly give them over to the butcher's knife? How could he or she devour their flesh as a sweet morsel?

It is a mistake to suppose that muscular strength depends on the use of animal food. The needs of the system can be better supplied, and more vigorous health can be enjoyed, without its use. Grains, with fruits, nuts, and vegetables, contain all the nutritive properties necessary to make good blood. These elements are not so well or so fully supplied by a flesh diet. Had the use of flesh been essential to health and strength, animal food would have been included in the diet appointed human beings in the beginning.

When the use of flesh food is discontinued, often there is a sense of weakness, a lack of vigor. Many urge this as evidence that flesh food is essential, but this is false reasoning. Flesh food is missed because it is stimulating; it fevers the blood and excites the nerves. Some will find it as difficult to leave off flesh eating as it is for drunkards to give up liquor, but they will be the better for the change.

When flesh food is discarded, its place should be supplied with a variety of grains, nuts, vegetables, and fruits that will be both nourishing and appetizing. This is especially necessary in the case of those who are weak or those who must do continual hard work. In some countries where poverty abounds, flesh is the cheapest food. Under these circumstances the change will be made with greater difficulty, but it can be done. We should, however, consider the situation of the people and the power of lifelong habit, being careful not to urge unduly even right ideas. None should be urged to make the change abruptly. The place of meat should be supplied with wholesome foods that are inexpensive. In this matter very much depends on the cook. With care and skill, dishes may be prepared that will be both nutritious and appetizing, and will, to a great degree, take the place of flesh food.

In all cases educate the conscience, enlist the will, and supply good, wholesome food. This will enable the change to be readily made, and the demand for flesh will soon cease.

Is it not time that all should aim to dispense with flesh foods? How can those who are seeking to become pure, refined, and holy, that they may have the companionship of heavenly angels, continue to use as food anything that has so harmful an effect on soul and body? How can they take the life of God's creatures that they may consume the flesh as a luxury? Let them, rather, return to the wholesome and delicious food given to the human race in the beginning. And let them practice, and teach their children to practice, mercy toward the dumb creatures that God has made and placed under our dominion.

C h a p t e r   2 5

Extremes
in Diet

Not all who profess to believe in diet reform are really reformers. With many the reform consists merely in discarding certain unwholesome foods. They do not understand clearly the principles of health. Their tables, still loaded with rich foods and delicacies, are far from being an example of Christian temperance and moderation.

Another class, in their desire to set a right example, go to the opposite extreme. If they are unable to obtain the most desirable foods, they adopt an impoverished diet instead of using such things as would best supply the lack. Their food does not supply the elements needed to make good blood. Their health suffers, their usefulness is impaired, and their example turns people against reform in diet.

Others think that since health requires a simple diet, one need give little thought to choosing or preparing food. Some restrict themselves to a very meager diet that lacks enough variety to supply the needs of the system, and they suffer in consequence.

Those who have but a partial understanding of the principles of reform are often the most rigid, not only in carrying out their views themselves but in urging them on their families and their neighbors. The effect of their mistaken reforms, as seen in their own ill health and their efforts to force their views upon others, give many a false idea of reform in diet and lead them to reject it altogether.

Those who understand the laws of health and who are governed by principle shun both the extremes of indulgence and of restriction. Their diet is chosen, not for the mere gratification of appetite, but for the upbuilding of the body. They seek to preserve every power in the best condition for highest service to God and man. Appetite is under the control of reason and conscience, and they are rewarded with health of body and mind. They do not urge their views offensively upon others, but their example is a testimony in favor of right principles. These persons have a wide influence for good.

There is real common sense in diet reform. The subject should be studied broadly and deeply, and we should not criticize others because their practice is not, in all things, in harmony with our own. It is impossible to make an unvarying rule to regulate everyone's habits, and we should not use ourselves as a criterion for all. Not all can eat the same things. Foods that are palatable and wholesome to one person may be distasteful, even harmful, to another. Some cannot use milk, while others thrive on it. Some persons cannot digest peas and beans; others find them wholesome. For some the coarser grain preparations are good food, while others cannot use them.

Those who live in new countries or in poverty-stricken districts, where fruits and nuts are scarce, should not be urged to exclude milk and eggs from their daily diet. It is true that robust persons in whom the animal passions are strong need to avoid the use of stimulating foods. Especially in families of children who are given to sensual habits, eggs should not be used. But in the case of persons whose blood-making organs are feeble— especially if other foods to supply the needed elements cannot be obtained— milk and eggs should not be wholly discarded. Great care should be taken, however, to obtain milk from healthy cows and eggs from healthy fowls that are well fed and well cared for; and the eggs should be so cooked as to be most easily digested.

Reform Should Be Progressive

The diet reform should be progressive. As disease in animals increases, the use of milk and eggs will become more and more unsafe. An effort should be made to supply their place with other things that are healthful and inexpensive. The people everywhere should be taught how to cook without milk and eggs, so far as possible, and yet have their food wholesome and palatable.

The practice of eating only two meals a day is generally found to be beneficial to health, yet under some circumstances persons may require a third meal. But, if taken at all, this should be very light, and of food most easily digested. "Crackers"—the English biscuit—or zwieback, plus fruit or a non-caffeinated drink made from grain, are the foods best suited for the evening meal.

Some continually fear that their food, however simple and healthful, may hurt them. To these let me say, Do not think that your food will injure you. Do not think about it at all. Eat according to your best judgment, and when you have asked the Lord to bless the food for the strengthening of your body, believe that He hears your prayer. Then relax and be at rest.

Principle requires us to discard those things that irritate the stomach and impair health, but we should remember that an impoverished diet produces poverty of the blood. Cases of disease most difficult to cure result from this cause. The system is not sufficiently nourished, and chronic indigestion and general debility are the result. Those who use such a diet are not always compelled by poverty to do so, but they choose it through ignorance or negligence, or to carry out their erroneous ideas of reform.

Eat Well to Keep Well

God is not honored when the body is neglected or abused and is thus unfitted for His service. To care for the body by providing for it food that is relishable and strengthening is one of the first duties of the householder. It is far better to have less expensive clothing and furniture than to stint on the supply of food.

Some householders stint the family table in order to entertain visitors lavishly. This is unwise. In the entertainment of guests there should be greater simplicity. Let the needs of the family have first attention.

Unwise economy and artificial customs often prevent the exercise of hospitality where it is needed and would be a blessing. The regular supply of food for our tables should be such that the unexpected guest can be made welcome without burdening the housewife to make extra preparation.

All should learn what to eat and how to cook. Men, as well as women, need to understand the simple, healthful preparation of food. If they have a knowledge of cookery, they can use it to good purpose when their business calls them where they cannot obtain wholesome food.

Carefully consider your diet. Study from cause to effect. Cultivate self-control. Keep appetite under the control of reason. Never abuse the stomach by overeating, but do not deprive yourself of the wholesome, palatable food that health demands.

The narrow ideas of some would-be health reformers have been a great injury to the cause of healthful living. Those who advocate the principles of healthful living should remember that reform in diet will be judged, to a great degree, by the provision they make for their tables; and they should so exemplify its principles as to commend them to candid minds. There is a large class who will oppose any reform movement, however reasonable, if it places a restriction on the appetite. They consult taste instead of reason or the laws of health. This class will consider as radical all who advocate reform, no matter how consistent their course. That these persons may have no ground for criticism, health reformers should not try to see how different they can be from others, but should come as near to them as possible without sacrificing principle.

When those who advocate reform in health practices go to extremes, it is no wonder that many who regard these persons as representing health principles reject the reform altogether. These extremes frequently do more harm in a short time than could be undone by a lifetime of consistent living.

True health reform is based upon principles that are broad and far-reaching, and we should not discredit it by narrow views and practices. Nor should we permit opposition or ridicule, or a desire to please or influence others, to turn us from true principles or cause us lightly to regard them. Those who are governed by principle will be firm and decided in standing for the right, yet in all their associations they will manifest a generous, Christlike spirit and true moderation.

Stimulants
and Narcotics

Under the heading of stimulants and narcotics is classed a great variety of substances that, when used as food or drink, irritate the stomach, poison the blood, and excite the nerves. Their use is a positive evil. People seek the excitement of stimulants because, for the time, the results are agreeable. But there is always a reaction. The use of unnatural stimulants always tends to excess, and it is an active agent in promoting physical degeneration and decay.

Condiments

In this fast age, the less exciting the food, the better. Condiments are injurious in their nature. Mustard, pepper, spices, pickles, and other things of like character irritate the stomach and make the blood feverish and impure. The inflamed condition of the drunkard's stomach is often pictured as illustrating the effect of alcoholic liquors. A similarly inflamed condition is produced by the use of irritating condiments. Soon ordinary food does not satisfy the appetite. The system feels a want, a craving, for something more stimulating.

Tea and Coffee

Tea acts as a stimulant and, to a certain extent, produces intoxication. The action of coffee and many other popular drinks is similar. The first effect is exhilarating. The nerves of the stomach are excited. These convey irritation to the brain which, in turn, is aroused to impart increased action to the heart and short-lived energy to the entire system. Fatigue is forgotten. Strength seems to be increased. The intellect is aroused, and the imagination becomes more vivid.

Because of these results, many suppose that tea or coffee is doing them great good. But this is a mistake. Tea and coffee do not nourish the system. Their effect is produced before there has been time for digestion and assimilation. What seems to be strength is only nervous excitement. When the influence of the stimulant is gone, the unnatural force abates, and the result is a corresponding degree of weakness and listlessness.

The continued use of these nerve irritants is followed by headache, wakefulness, palpitation of the heart, indigestion, trembling, and many other evils, for they wear away the life forces. Tired nerves need rest and quiet instead of stimulation and overwork. Nature needs time to recuperate her exhausted energies. When her forces are goaded on by the use of stimulants, more will be accomplished for a time, but, as the system becomes debilitated by their constant use, it gradually becomes more difficult to rouse the energies to the desired point. The demand for stimulants becomes more difficult to control, until the will is overborne and there seems to be no power to deny the unnatural craving. Stronger and still stronger stimulants are called for, until exhausted nature can no longer respond.

The Tobacco Habit

Tobacco is a slow, insidious, but most malignant poison. In whatever form it is used, it affects one's constitution adversely. It is all the more dangerous because its effects are slow and at first hardly perceptible. It excites and then paralyzes the nerves. It weakens and clouds the brain. Often it affects the nerves in a more powerful manner than does intoxicating drink. It is more subtle, and its effects are difficult to eradicate from the system. Its use excites a thirst for strong drink and in many cases lays the foundation for the liquor habit.

The use of tobacco is inconvenient, expensive, uncleanly, defiling to the user, and offensive to others. Its devotees are encountered everywhere. You rarely pass through a crowd but some smoker puffs his poisoned breath in your face. It is unpleasant and unhealthful to remain in a railway car or in a room where the atmosphere is laden with the fumes of liquor and tobacco. Though people persist in using these poisons themselves, what right have they to defile the air that others must breathe?*

Among children and youth the use of tobacco is working untold harm. The unhealthful practices of past generations affect the children and youth of today. Mental inability, physical weakness, disordered nerves, and un-

---

* Many countries have now passed laws that forbid smoking in public buildings, railway cars, buses, and airplanes.—Publisher.

natural cravings are transmitted as a legacy from parents to children. And the same practices, continued by the children, are increasing and perpetuating the evil results. To no small degree this is the cause of the physical, mental, and moral deterioration that is becoming such a cause of alarm.

Boys begin the use of tobacco at a very early age. The habit thus formed when body and mind are especially susceptible to its effects undermines the physical strength, dwarfs the body, stupefies the mind, and corrupts the morals.

But what can be done to teach children and youth the evils of a practice of which parents, teachers, and ministers set them the example? Little boys, hardly emerged from babyhood, may be seen smoking cigarettes. If one speaks to them about it, they say, "My father uses tobacco." They point to the minister or the Sunday-school superintendent and say, "Such a man smokes; what harm for me to do as he does?" Many workers in the temperance cause are addicted to the use of tobacco. What power can such persons have to stay the progress of intemperance?

I appeal to those who profess to believe and obey the Word of God: Can you as Christians indulge a habit that is paralyzing your intellect and robbing you of power rightly to estimate eternal realities? Can you consent daily to rob God of service that is His due, and to rob other people both of service you might render and of the power of example?

As God's stewards, have you considered your responsibility for the means in your hands? How much of the Lord's money do you spend for tobacco? Add up what you have spent during your lifetime. How does the amount consumed by this defiling lust compare with what you have given for the relief of the poor and the spread of the gospel?

No human being needs tobacco, but multitudes are perishing for want of the means that by its use is worse than wasted. Have you not been misappropriating the Lord's goods? Have you not been guilty of robbery toward God and needy people? "Do you not know that . . . you are not your own? For you were bought at a price; therefore glorify God in your body and in your spirit, which are God's." 1 Corinthians 6:19, 20.

Intoxicating Drinks

"Wine is a mocker, intoxicating drink arouses brawling,
And whoever is led astray by it is not wise."
"Who has woe?
Who has sorrow?
Who has contentions?
Who has complaints?
Who has wounds without cause?
Who has redness of eyes?
Those who linger long at the wine,

Those who go in search of mixed wine.
Do not look on the wine when it is red,
When it sparkles in the cup,
When it swirls around smoothly;
At the last it bites like a serpent,
And stings like a viper."
Proverbs 20:1; 23:29-32.

Never was traced by human hand a more vivid picture of the debasement and slavery of victims of intoxicating drink. Enthralled, degraded, even when awakened to a sense of their misery these victims have no power to break from the snare; they will "seek another drink." Proverbs 23:35.

No argument is needed to show the evil effects of intoxicants on the drunkard. The bleared, besotted wrecks of humanity—souls for whom Christ died and over whom angels weep—are everywhere. They are a blot on our boasted civilization. They are the shame and curse and peril of every land.

And who can picture the wretchedness, the agony, the despair, that are hidden in the drunkard's home? Think of the wife, often delicately reared, sensitive, cultured, and refined, linked to one whom drink transforms into a sot or a demon. Think of the children, robbed of home comforts, education, and training, living in terror of him who should be their pride and protection, thrust into the world, bearing the brand of shame, often with the hereditary curse of the drunkard's thirst.

Think of the frightful accidents that are every day occurring through the influence of drink. Some official on a railway train neglects to heed a signal or misinterprets an order. On goes the train. There is a collision, and many lives are lost. Or a ship runs aground, and passengers and crew find a watery grave. When the matter is investigated, it is found that someone at an important post was under the influence of drink. To what extent can one indulge the liquor habit and be safely trusted with the lives of human beings? Only one who totally abstains can be trusted.

The Milder Intoxicants

Persons who have inherited an appetite for unnatural stimulants should by no means have wine, beer, or cider in their sight or within their reach, for this keeps the temptation constantly before them. Regarding sweet cider as harmless, many have no scruples in purchasing it freely. But it remains sweet for a short time only; then fermentation begins. The sharp taste that it then acquires makes it all the more acceptable to many palates, and the user is loath to admit that it has become hard, or fermented.

There is danger to health in the use of even sweet cider as ordinarily produced. If people could see what the microscope reveals in regard to the cider they buy, few would be willing to drink it. Often those who manufacture cider for the market are not careful as to the condition of the fruit squeezed, sometimes including even wormy or decayed apples. Those who would not think of using the poisonous, rotten apples in any other way will drink the cider made from them and call it a luxury; but the microscope shows that even when fresh from the press, this pleasant beverage is wholly unfit for use.*

Intoxication is just as really produced by wine, beer, and cider as by stronger drinks. The use of these drinks awakens the taste for those that are stronger, and thus the liquor habit is established. Moderate drinking is the school in which people are educated to be drunkards. Yet so insidious is the work of these milder stimulants that the highway to drunkenness is entered before the victim suspects danger.

Some who are never considered really drunk are always under the influence of mild intoxicants. They are feverish, unstable in mind, unbalanced. Imagining themselves secure, they go on and on until every barrier is broken down, every principle sacrificed, the strongest resolutions undermined. The highest considerations are not sufficient to keep the debased appetite under the control of reason.

The Bible nowhere sanctions the use of intoxicating wine. The wine that Christ made from water at the marriage feast of Cana was the pure juice of the grape. This is "'the new wine . . . found in the cluster,'" of which the Scripture says, "'"Do not destroy it, for a blessing is in it."'" Isaiah 65:8.

It was Christ who, in the Old Testament, gave the warning to Israel, "Wine is a mocker, intoxicating drink arouses brawling, and whoever is led astray by it is not wise." Proverbs 20:1.

He Himself provided no such beverage. Satan tempts people to indulgence that will becloud reason and benumb the spiritual perceptions, but Christ teaches us to bring the lower nature into subjection. He never places before us that which would be a temptation. His whole life was an example of self-denial. It was to break the power of appetite that in the forty days' fast in the wilderness He suffered in our behalf the severest test that humanity could endure.

It was Christ who directed that John the Baptist should drink neither wine nor strong drink. It was He who enjoined similar abstinence upon the wife of Manoah.

Christ did not contradict His own teaching. The unfermented wine that He provided for the wedding guests was a wholesome and refreshing drink. This is the wine that was used by our Savior and His disciples in the first

---

* When the author wrote this in 1905, it was common practice to manufacture cider as here described. But today where cider is produced under sanitary conditions, using good, sound fruit, this comment may not be applicable.—Publisher.

Communion. It is the wine that should always be used on the Communion table as a symbol of the Savior's blood. The sacramental service is designed to be soul-refreshing and life-giving. Nothing is to be connected with it that could minister to evil.

In the light of what the Scriptures, nature, and reason teach concerning the use of intoxicants, how can Christians engage in the raising of hops for beer making? How can they engage in the manufacture of wine or cider for the market? If they love their neighbors as themselves, how can they help to place in their way that which will be a snare to them?

Often intemperance begins in the home. By the use of rich, unhealthful food the digestive organs are weakened and a desire is created for food that is stimulating. Thus the appetite is educated to crave something still stronger. The demand for stimulants becomes more frequent and more difficult to resist. The system becomes more or less filled with poison, and the more debilitated it becomes, the greater is the desire for these things. One step in the wrong direction prepares the way for another. Many who would not be guilty of placing on their table wine or liquor will load their table with food that creates such a thirst for strong drink that to resist the temptation is almost impossible. Wrong habits of eating and drinking destroy the health and prepare the way for drunkenness.

There would soon be little necessity for temperance campaigns if right principles in regard to temperance could be implanted in the youth who form and fashion society. Let parents conduct a campaign against intemperance at their own firesides, in the principles they teach their children to follow from infancy, and they may hope for success.

There is work for mothers in helping their children to form correct habits and pure tastes. Educate the appetite; teach the children to abhor stimulants. Bring your children up to have moral stamina to resist the evil that surrounds them. Teach them that they are not to be swayed by others, that they are not to yield to evil influences, however strong, but to influence others for good.

Great efforts are made to put down intemperance, but there is much effort that is not directed to the right point. The advocates of temperance reform should be awake to the evils resulting from the use of unwholesome food, condiments, tea, and coffee. We wish temperance workers the best of success; but we invite them to look more deeply into the causes of the evil they war against and to be sure they are consistent in reform.

It must be kept before the people that the right balance of the mental and moral powers depends in a great degree on the right condition of the physical system. All narcotics and unnatural stimulants that enfeeble and degrade the physical nature tend to lower the tone of the intellect and morals. Intemperance lies at the foundation of the moral depravity of the world. By the indulgence of perverted appetite, people lose their power to resist temptation.

Temperance reformers have a work to do in educating their hearers along these lines. Teach them that health, character, and even life are endangered by the use of stimulants, which excite the exhausted energies to unnatural, spasmodic action.

In relation to tea, coffee, tobacco, and alcoholic drinks, the only safe course is to touch not, taste not, handle not. The tendency of tea, coffee, and similar drinks is in the same direction as that of liquor and tobacco, and in some cases the habit is as difficult to break as it is for the alcoholic to give up intoxicants.

Those who attempt to leave off these stimulants will for a time feel a loss and will suffer without them. But by persistence they will overcome the craving and cease to feel the lack. Nature may require a little time to recover from the abuse she has suffered, but give her a chance and she will again rally and perform her work nobly and well.

Chapter 27

Evils of the Drug and Liquor Traffic

"'Woe to him who builds his house by unrighteousness and his chambers by injustice, . . . who says, "I will build myself a wide house with spacious chambers, and cut out windows for it, paneling it with cedar and painting it with vermilion." Shall you reign because you enclose yourself in cedar? . . . Your eyes and your heart are for nothing but your covetousness, for shedding innocent blood, and practicing oppression and violence.'" Jeremiah 22:13-17.

This scripture pictures the work of those who manufacture and who sell intoxicating liquor. Their business means robbery. For the money they receive, no equivalent is returned. Every dollar they add to their gains brings a curse to the spender.

With a liberal hand, God has bestowed His blessings upon the human family. If His gifts were wisely used, the world would know little of poverty or distress! But wickedness has turned His blessings into a curse. Through greed of gain and the lust of appetite, the grains and fruits given for our sustenance are converted into poisons that bring misery and ruin.

Every year millions and millions of gallons of intoxicating liquors are consumed. Millions upon millions of dollars are spent to buy wretchedness, poverty, disease, degradation, lust, crime, and death. For the sake of gain, the liquor dealer sells that which corrupts and destroys mind and body. He entails on the drunkard's family poverty and wretchedness.

When his victim is dead, he does not hesitate to take the very necessities of life from the destitute family, to pay the drink bill of the husband

and father. The cries of the suffering children, the tears of the widowed mother only exasperate him. He grows rich on the misery of those whom he is leading to perdition.

To a great degree, prostitution, vice, violent crimes, and poverty are a result of the liquor seller's work. Like the mystic Babylon of the Apocalypse, he is dealing in "bodies and souls of men." Behind the liquor seller stands the mighty destroyer of souls, and every art that earth or hell can devise is employed to draw human beings under his power. In the city and the country, on the railway trains, on the great steamers, in places of business, in the halls of pleasure, in the medical dispensary, even in the church on the sacred Communion table, his traps are set. Nothing is left undone to create and to foster the desire for intoxicants. On corner after corner stand taverns or night clubs, with their brilliant lights, welcome, and good cheer, inviting the working man, the wealthy idler, and the unsuspecting youth.

In private lunchrooms and fashionable resorts, women are supplied with popular drinks containing alcohol. For the sick and the exhausted, there are the widely advertised tonics, consisting largely of alcohol.

To create the liquor appetite in little children, alcohol is introduced into confectionery. Such confectionery is sold in the shops. And by the gift of these candies the liquor seller entices children into his resorts.

Day by day, month by month, year by year, the work goes on. Fathers and husbands and brothers, the hope and pride of the nation, are steadily passing into the liquor dealer's haunts, to be wrecked and ruined.

More terrible still, the curse is striking the very heart of the home. More and more women are forming the liquor habit. In many a household, little children, even in the innocence and helplessness of babyhood, are in daily peril through the neglect, abuse, and vileness of drunken mothers. Sons and daughters are growing up under the shadow of this terrible evil. What outlook for their future but that they will sink even lower than their parents?

From so-called Christian lands the curse is carried to developing nations. The poor and ignorant are taught the use of liquor. Men and women of intelligence recognize and protest against it as a deadly poison, but their efforts to protect their lands from its ravages have been in vain. By civilized peoples, tobacco, liquor, and opium are forced upon various nations. The ungoverned passions of the people, stimulated by drink, drag them down to degradation unknown before, and it becomes an almost hopeless undertaking to send messengers of the gospel to these lands.

Through their contact with peoples who should have given them a knowledge of God, pagans and idolaters are led into vices that are proving the destruction of whole tribes and races. And in the dark places of the earth the representatives of civilized nations are hated because of this.

The Responsibility of the Church

The liquor interest is a power in the world. It has on its side the combined strength of money, habit, appetite. Its power is felt even in the church. People whose money has been made, directly or indirectly, in the liquor traffic are members of churches "in good and regular standing." Many of them give liberally to popular charities. Their contributions help to support the enterprises of the church and to sustain its ministers. They command the consideration shown to the power of money. Churches that accept such members are virtually sustaining the liquor traffic. Too often ministers do not have the courage to stand for the right. They do not declare to their people what God has said concerning the work of the liquor seller. To speak plainly would mean offending the congregation, sacrificing popularity, and losing income.

But above the tribunal of the church is the tribunal of God. He who declared to the first murderer, "'The voice of your brother's blood cries out to Me from the ground'" (Genesis 4:10), will not accept for His altar the gifts of the liquor dealer. His anger is kindled against those who attempt to cover their guilt with a cloak of liberality. Their money is stained with blood. A curse is upon it.

> "'To what purpose is the multitude of your sacrifices
>   to Me?' says the Lord. . . .
> 'When you come to appear before Me,
> Who has required this from your hand, to trample My courts?
> Bring no more futile sacrifices. . . .
> When you spread out your hands,
> I will hide My eyes from you;
> Even though you make many prayers, I will not hear.
> Your hands are full of blood.'"
>
> Isaiah 1:11-15.

Drunkards are capable of better things. They have been entrusted with talents with which to honor God and bless the world, but fellow humans have laid a snare for their souls. They have built themselves up by degrading others, living in luxury while the poor victims whom they have robbed live in poverty and wretchedness. But God will call to account those who helped speed drunkards to ruin. He who rules in the heavens has not lost sight of the first cause or the last effect of drunkenness. He who cares for the sparrow and clothes the grass of the field will not pass by those who have been formed in His own image, purchased with His own blood. He will heed their cries. God marks all this wickedness that perpetuates crime and misery.

The world and the church may have approval for the person who has gained wealth by degrading the human soul. They may smile upon the one by whom men and women are led down step by step in the path of shame and degradation. But God notes it all and renders a just judgment. The liquor seller may be termed by the world a good businessman, but the Lord says, "Woe unto him." He will be charged with the hopelessness, the misery, the suffering, brought into the world by the liquor traffic. He will have to answer for the want and woe of the mothers and children who have suffered for lack of food and clothing and shelter and who have buried all hope and joy. He will have to answer for the souls he has sent unprepared into eternity. And those who sustain the liquor seller in his work are sharers in his guilt. To them God says, "Your hands are full of blood."

License Laws

The licensing of the liquor traffic, it is argued, tends to restrict its evil. But the licensing of the traffic places it under the protection of law. The government sanctions its existence and thus fosters the evil that it professes to restrict. Under the protection of license laws, breweries, distilleries, and wineries are operating all over the land, and the liquor seller carries on his work beside our very doors.

Often he is forbidden to sell intoxicants to one who is drunk or who is known to be a confirmed drunkard, but the work of leading youth to become drunkards goes steadily forward. The very life of the traffic depends upon creating the liquor appetite in youth. The youth are led on, step by step, until the liquor habit is established and the thirst is created that at any cost demands satisfaction. It would be less harmful to grant liquor to the confirmed drunkard, whose ruin, in most cases, is already determined, than to permit our youth to be lured to destruction through this terrible habit.

By licensing the liquor traffic, temptation is kept constantly before those who are trying to reform. Institutions have been established where the victims of intemperance may be helped to overcome their appetite. This is a noble work, but as long as the sale of liquor is sanctioned by law, the intemperate receive little benefit from these institutions. They cannot remain there always. They must again take their place in society. The appetite for intoxicating drink, though subdued, is not wholly destroyed, and when temptation assails them, as it does on every hand, they too often fall an easy prey.

A person who has a vicious beast and who, knowing its disposition, allows it unrestricted freedom is by the laws of the land held accountable for the evil the beast may do. In the laws given to Israel the Lord directed that when a beast known to be vicious caused the death of a human being, the life of the owner should pay the price of his carelessness or intention to harm others. On the same principle the government that licenses the liquor seller should be held responsible for the results of his traffic. And if it is a crime worthy of death to let a vicious beast kill someone, how much greater is the crime of sanctioning the work of the liquor seller!

The argument for granting licenses is that they bring revenue into the public treasury. But what is this revenue when compared with the enormous expense incurred for the criminals, the insane, the extremely poor, that are the fruit of the liquor traffic!

A person under the influence of liquor commits a serious crime and is brought into court. Those who legalized the traffic are forced to deal with the result of their own work. They authorized the sale of an intoxicating drink, and now it is necessary for them to sentence the person to prison or to death, while often the family is left in financial straits, dependent on church or civic organizations.

Considering only the financial aspect of the question, it is irrational to tolerate such a business! But what revenue can compensate for the loss of human reason, for defacing the image of God in a person, for ruining children, reducing them to pauperism and degradation, and often perpetuating in them the evil tendencies of drunken parents?

People who have formed the habit of using intoxicants are in a desperate situation. Their brains are diseased, their will power weakened. Without divine help, their appetite is uncontrollable. They cannot be reasoned with or persuaded to deny themselves. When in the company of others who are drinking, a person who has resolved to quit is led to pick up the glass again, and with the first taste of the intoxicant every good resolution is overpowered. One taste of the liquor, and all thought of its results vanishes. The faithful spouse is forgotten. The children may be hungry and without clothes, but that no longer matters. By legalizing the traffic, the law gives its sanction to this downfall of the soul and refuses to stop the trade that fills the world with evil.

Must this always continue? Will souls always have to struggle for victory, with the door of temptation wide open before them? Must the curse of intemperance forever rest like a blight upon the civilized world? Must it continue to sweep, every year, like a devouring fire over thousands of happy homes? When a ship is wrecked in sight of shore, people do not idly look on. They risk their lives in an effort to rescue men and women from a watery grave. How much greater the demand for effort in rescuing them from the alcoholic's fate!

We are all woven together in the web of humanity. The evil that befalls any part of the great human family brings peril to all.

Many men and women who through love of gain or ease would have nothing to do with restricting the liquor traffic have found, too late, that the traffic had a terrible impact on them. They have seen their own children become alcoholics and ruined. Lawlessness runs riot. Property is in danger. Life is unsafe. Accidents by sea and by land multiply. Diseases that breed in an environment of filth and wretchedness make their way to lordly and luxurious homes. Vices fostered by the children of debauchery and crime infect the sons and daughters of refined and cultured households.

There is no one whose interests the liquor traffic does not imperil. There is no one who should not do everything possible to destroy it.

Above all other places having to do with secular interests only, legislative halls and courts of justice should be free from the curse of intemperance. Governors, senators, representatives, judges, people who enact and administer a nation's laws, people who hold in their hands the lives, the reputation, the possessions of other humans, should be persons of strict temperance. Only thus can their minds be clear to discriminate between right and wrong. Only thus can they possess firmness of principle and wisdom to administer justice and show mercy.

But how does the record stand? Many of these authority figures have their minds beclouded, their sense of right and wrong confused, by strong drink. Many are the oppressive laws enacted, many the innocent persons condemned to death through the injustice of drinking lawmakers, witnesses, jurors, lawyers, and even judges. Many there are, "mighty at drinking wine," and "men valiant for mixing intoxicating drink," "who call evil good, and good evil," "who justify the wicked for a bribe, and take away justice from the righteous man." Of such God says:

"As the fire devours the stubble,
And the flame consumes the chaff,
So their root will be as rottenness,
And their blossom will ascend like dust;
Because they have rejected the law of the Lord of hosts,
And despised the word of the Holy One of Israel."
                                        Isaiah 5:20-24.

The honor of God, the stability of the nation, the well-being of the community, of the home, and of the individual, demand that every possible effort be made to arouse the people to the evil of intemperance. Soon we shall see the result of this terrible evil as we do not see it now. Who will put forth a determined effort to halt the work of destruction? As yet the contest has hardly begun. Let an army be formed to stop the sale of the drugs and liquors that are making people mad. Let the danger from the liquor traffic be made plain and a public sentiment be created that shall demand its prohibition. Let drunks and alcoholics be given an opportunity to escape from their thralldom. Let the voice of the nation demand of its lawmakers that a stop be put to this infamous traffic.

"Deliver those who are drawn toward death,
And hold back those stumbling to the slaughter.
If you say, 'Surely we did not know this,'
Does not He who weighs the hearts consider it?
He who keeps your soul, does He not know it?"
"What will you say when He punishes you?"
            Proverbs 24:11, 12; Jeremiah 13:21.

The Home

$\mathcal{C} h a p t e r \quad 28$

Ministry of the Home

Restoring and uplifting humanity begins in the home. The work of parents underlies every other. Society is composed of families and is what the heads of families make it. Out of the heart "spring the issues of life" (Proverbs 4:23). The heart of the community, of the church, and of the nation is the household. The well-being of society, the success of the church, the prosperity of the nation depend upon home influences.

The importance and the opportunities of home life are illustrated in the life of Jesus. He who came from heaven to be our example and teacher spent thirty years as a member of the household at Nazareth. Concerning these years the Bible record is very brief. No mighty miracles attracted the attention of the multitude. No eager throngs followed Jesus' steps or listened to His words. Yet during all those years He was fulfilling His divine mission. He lived as one of us, sharing the home life, submitting to its discipline, performing its duties, bearing its burdens. In the sheltering care of a humble home, participating in the experiences of our common lot, He "increased in wisdom and stature, and in favor with God and men." Luke 2:52.

During all these secluded years His life flowed out in currents of sympathy and helpfulness. His unselfishness and patient endurance, His courage and faithfulness, His resistance of temptation, His unfailing peace and quiet joyfulness were a constant inspiration. He brought a pure, sweet atmosphere into the home, and His life was as leaven working amidst the elements of society. No one said that He had performed a miracle, yet virtue—the healing, life-giving power of love—went out from Him to the tempted, the sick, and the disheartened. In an unobtrusive way, even from childhood, Jesus ministered to others, and because of this, when He began His public ministry, many heard Him gladly.

The Savior's early years are not only an example to youth, they are a lesson, and should be an encouragement, to every parent. The circle of family and neighborhood duties is the very first field of effort for those who would work to improve society. There is no more important field of effort than that committed to the founders and guardians of the home. No work entrusted to human beings involves greater or more far-reaching results than does the work of fathers and mothers.

By the youth and children of today the future of society is determined, and what these youth and children shall be depends upon the home. To the lack of right home training may be traced the larger share of the disease, misery, and crime that curse humanity. If the home life were pure and true, if the children who went forth from its care were prepared to meet life's responsibilities and dangers, what a change would be seen in the world!

Great efforts are put forth, time and money and labor almost without limit are expended, in enterprises and institutions for reforming the victims of evil habits. And even these efforts are inadequate to meet the great necessity. Small is the result, and few victims are permanently reclaimed.

Multitudes long for a better life, but they lack courage and resolution to break away from the power of habit. They shrink from the struggle and sacrifice demanded, and their lives are wrecked and ruined. Thus even people with the brightest minds, people of high aspirations and noble powers, who otherwise are fitted by nature and education to fill positions of trust and responsibility, are degraded and lost for this life and for the life to come.

Of those who do reform, many reap the harvest of their evil sowing all their life in a shattered physical constitution, a wavering will, impaired intellect, and weakened soul power. How much more might be accomplished if the evil were dealt with at the beginning!

The Responsibility of Parents

This work rests, in a great degree, on parents. Intemperance and other evils are eating like a cancer in the social body, but if more attention were given to teaching parents how to form the habits and character of their children, a hundredfold more good would result. It is in their power to make habit, which is so terrible a force for evil, into a force for good. Dealing with the stream at its source, it rests with them to direct it rightly.

Parents may lay for their children the foundation for a healthy, happy life. They may send them forth from their homes with moral stamina to resist temptation, and courage and strength to wrestle successfully with life's problems. They may inspire in them the purpose and develop the power to make their lives an honor to God and a blessing to the world. They may make straight paths for their feet, through sunshine and shadow, to the glorious heights above.

The mission of the home extends beyond its own members. The Christian home is to be an object lesson, illustrating the excellence of the true principles of life. Such an illustration will be a power for good in the world. Far more powerful than any sermon that can be preached is the influence of a true home upon human hearts and lives. As the youth go out from such a home, the lessons they have learned are shared with others. Nobler principles of life are introduced into other households, and an uplifting influence works in the community.

We might make our homes a blessing to many others. Our social entertainments should not be governed by the dictates of worldly custom but by the Spirit of Christ and the teaching of His Word. The Israelites, in all their festivities, included not only the poor and the stranger, but the Levite, who was both the assistant of the priest in the sanctuary and a religious teacher and missionary. These were regarded as the guests of the people, to share their hospitality on all occasions of social and religious rejoicing, and to be tenderly cared for when sick or in need. Persons such as these we should make welcome to our homes. How much such a welcome might do to cheer and encourage the missionary nurse or the teacher, the care-burdened, hard-working mother, or the feeble and aged, struggling with poverty and many discouragements.

"'When you give a dinner or a supper,'" Christ says, "'do not ask your friends, your brothers, your relatives, nor rich neighbors, lest they also invite you back, and you be repaid. But when you give a feast, invite the poor, the maimed, the lame, the blind. And you will be blessed, because they cannot repay you; for you shall be repaid at the resurrection of the just.'" Luke 14:12-14.

These are guests who will be no great burden to receive. You will not need to provide elaborate or expensive entertainment. You will not need to make an effort at display. To many of these people the warmth of a genial welcome, a place at your fireside, a seat at your home table, the privilege of sharing the blessing of the hour of prayer, would be like a glimpse of heaven.

Homes to Be a Blessing

Our sympathies are to overflow the boundaries of self and the enclosure of family walls. There are precious opportunities for those who will make their homes a blessing to others. Social influence is a wonderful power. We can use it as a means of helping those about us.

Our homes should be a place of refuge for tempted young people. Many are standing at the parting of the ways. Every influence, every impression, is determining the choice that shapes their present and eternal destiny. Evil invites them. Its resorts are bright and attractive. They welcome every comer. All about us are youth who have no home, and many whose homes have no helpful, uplifting power. Drifting into evil, these youth are going down to ruin within the very shadow of our own doors.

Stretch out a hand to them in sympathy. Kind words simply spoken, little attentions simply bestowed, will sweep away the clouds of temptation that gather over the soul. The true expression of heaven-born sympathy has power to open the door of hearts that need the fragrance of Christlike words and the simple, delicate touch of the spirit of Christ's love. If we would show an interest in the young people, invite them to our homes, and surround them with cheering, helpful influences, many would gladly turn their steps into the upward path.

Our time here is short. We pass through this world but once. Let us make the most of life. The work to which we are called does not require wealth or social position or great ability. It requires a kindly, self-sacrificing spirit and a steadfast purpose. A lamp, however small, if kept burning steadily, may be the means of lighting many other lamps. Our sphere of influence may seem narrow, our ability small, our opportunities few, our acquirements limited, yet wonderful possibilities are ours through a faithful use of the opportunities of our own homes. If we will open our hearts and homes to the divine principles of life, we shall become channels for currents of life-giving power. From our homes will flow streams of healing, bringing life and beauty and fruitfulness where now are barrenness and dearth.

Chapter 29

Builders
of the Home

At a marriage festival where friends and relatives rejoiced together, Christ began His public ministry by performing His first miracle. Thus He sanctioned marriage, recognizing it as an institution that He Himself had established. He ordained that men and women should be united in holy wedlock, to rear families whose members, crowned with honor, should be recognized as members of the family above.

Christ honored the marriage relation by also making it a symbol of the union between Him and His redeemed ones. He Himself is the Bridegroom; the bride is the church, of which, as His chosen one, He says, "'You are all fair, my love, and there is no spot in you.'" Song of Solomon 4:7.

Christ "loved the church and gave Himself for it, that He might sanctify and cleanse it . . . that it should be holy and without blemish. So husbands ought to love their own wives." Ephesians 5:25-28.

The family tie is the closest, the most tender and sacred, of any on earth. It was designed to be a blessing. And it is a blessing wherever the marriage covenant is entered into intelligently, in the fear of God, and with due consideration for its responsibilities.

Those who are contemplating marriage should consider what will be the character and influence of the home they are founding. As they become parents, a sacred trust is committed to them. Upon them depends in a great measure the well-being of their children in this world and their happiness in the world to come. To a great extent they determine both the physical and moral stamp that their little ones receive. And upon the character of the home depends the condition of society. Each family's influence helps either to elevate it or degrade it.

The choice of a life companion should be such as best to secure physical, mental, and spiritual well-being for parents and for their children—such as will enable both parents and children to bless other people and honor their Creator.

Before assuming the responsibilities involved in marriage, young men and young women should have such an experience in practical life as will prepare them for its duties and burdens. Early marriages should not be encouraged. A relation as important as marriage and so far-reaching in its results should not be entered upon hastily, without sufficient preparation and before the mental and physical powers are well developed.

The parties may not have worldly wealth, but they should have the far greater blessing of health. And in most cases they should not be far apart in age. A neglect of this rule may result in seriously impairing the health of the younger. And often the children are robbed of physical and mental strength. They cannot receive from an aged parent the care and companionship that their young lives demand, and they may be deprived by death of the father or the mother at the very time when love and guidance are most needed.

Only in Christ can a marriage alliance be safely formed. Human love should draw its closest bonds from divine love. Only where Christ reigns can there be deep, true, unselfish affection.

Love Is a Principle

Love is a precious gift that we receive from Jesus. Pure and holy affection is not a feeling but a principle. Those who are actuated by true love are neither unreasonable nor blind. Taught by the Holy Spirit, they love God supremely and their neighbor as themselves.

Let those who are contemplating marriage weigh every sentiment and watch every development of character in the one with whom they think to unite their life destiny. Let every step toward a marriage alliance be characterized by modesty, simplicity, sincerity, and an earnest purpose to please and honor God. Marriage affects the life of the couple both in this world and in the world to come. A sincere Christian will make no plans that God cannot approve.

If you are blessed with God-fearing parents, seek counsel of them. Open to them your hopes and plans, learn the lessons that their life experiences have taught, and you will be saved many a heartache. Above all, make Christ your counselor. Study His Word with prayer.

Under such guidance let a young woman accept as a life companion only one who possesses pure, manly traits of character, one who is diligent, aspiring, and honest, one who loves and fears God. Let a young man seek one to stand by his side who is fitted to bear her share of life's burdens, one whose influence will ennoble and refine him, and who will make him happy in her love.

"A prudent wife is from the Lord." "The heart of her husband safely trusts her. . . . She does him good and not evil all the days of her life." "She opens her mouth with wisdom, and on her tongue is the law of kindness. She watches over the ways of her household, and does not eat the bread of idleness. Her children rise up and call her blessed; her husband also, and he praises her," saying, "'Many daughters have done well, but you excel them all.'" "He who finds [such] a wife finds a good thing, and obtains favor from the Lord." Proverbs 19:14; 31:11, 12, 26-29; 18:22.

However carefully and wisely marriage may have been entered into, few couples are completely united when the marriage ceremony is performed. The real union of the two in wedlock is the work of the years that follow.

As life with its burden of perplexity and care meets the newly wedded pair, the romance with which imagination so often invests marriage disappears. Husband and wife learn each other's character as it was impossible to learn it in their previous association. This is a most critical period in their experience. Their happiness and usefulness in future years depend upon their taking a right course now. Often they discern in each other unsuspected weaknesses and defects, but the hearts that love has united will also discern excellencies unseen before. Let all seek to discover the excellencies rather than the defects.

Often it is our own attitude, the atmosphere that surrounds ourselves, that determines what will be revealed to us in another. There are many who regard the expression of love as a weakness, and they maintain a reserve that repels others. This spirit checks the current of sympathy. As the social and generous impulses are repressed, they wither, and the heart becomes desolate and cold. We should beware of this error. Love cannot long exist without expression. Let not the heart of one connected with you starve for the want of kindness and sympathy.

Though difficulties, perplexities, and discouragements may arise, let neither husband nor wife harbor the thought that their union is a mistake or a disappointment. Determine to be all that it is possible to be to each other. Continue the early attentions. In every way encourage each other in fighting the battles of life. Study to advance the happiness of the other. Let there be mutual love, mutual forbearance. Then marriage, instead of being the end of love, will be, as it were, the very beginning of love. The warmth of true friendship, the love that binds heart to heart, is a foretaste of the joys of heaven.

Around every family there is a sacred circle that should be kept unbroken. Within this circle no other person has a right to come. Let not the husband or the wife permit another to share the confidences that belong solely to themselves.

Let each give love rather than exact it. Cultivate that which is noblest in yourselves, and be quick to recognize the good qualities in the other. The consciousness of being appreciated is a wonderful stimulus and satisfaction. Sympathy and respect encourage one to strive toward excellence, and love itself increases as it stimulates to nobler aims.

Neither the husband nor the wife should merge his or her individuality in that of the other. Each has a personal relation to God. Of Him each is to ask, "What is right?" "What is wrong?" "How may I best fulfill life's purpose?" Let the wealth of your affection flow forth to Him who gave His life for you. Make Christ first and last and best in everything. As your love for Him becomes deeper and stronger, your love for each other will be purified and strengthened.

The spirit that Christ manifests toward us is the spirit that husband and wife are to manifest toward each other. "As Christ also has loved us," "walk in love." "As the church is subject to Christ, so let the wives be to their own husbands in everything. Husbands, love your wives, just as Christ also loved the church and gave Himself for it." Ephesians 5:2, 24, 25.

Neither the husband nor the wife should attempt to exercise arbitrary control over the other. Do not try to compel each other to yield to your wishes. You cannot do this and retain each other's love. Be kind, patient, and forbearing, considerate, and courteous. By the grace of God you can succeed in making each other happy, as in your marriage vow you promised to do.

Happiness in Unselfish Service

But remember that happiness will not be found in shutting yourselves up to yourselves, satisfied to pour out all your affection upon each other. Seize every opportunity to contribute to the happiness of those around you. Remember that true joy can be found only in unselfish service.

Forbearance and unselfishness mark the words and acts of all who live the new life in Christ. As you seek to live His life, striving to conquer self and selfishness and to minister to the needs of others, you will gain victory after victory. Thus your influence will bless the world.

Men and women can reach God's ideal for them if they will take Christ as their Helper. What human wisdom cannot do, His grace will accomplish for those who give themselves to Him in loving trust. His providence can unite hearts in bonds that are of heavenly origin. Love will not be a mere exchange of soft and flattering words. The loom of heaven weaves with warp and woof finer, yet more firm, than can be woven by the looms of earth. The result is not a delicate fabric but a texture that will bear wear and test and trial. Heart will be bound to heart in the golden bonds of a love that is enduring.

> Better than gold is a peaceful home,
> Where all the fireside charities come;
> The shrine of love and the heaven of life,
> Hallowed by mother, or sister, or wife.
> However humble the home may be,
> Or tried with sorrows by Heaven's decree,
> The blessings that never were bought or sold,
> And center there, are better than gold.
>
> Anon.

Chapter 30

Choice and Preparation of the Home

The gospel is a wonderful simplifier of life's problems. Its instruction, heeded, would make plain many a perplexity and save us from many an error. It teaches us to estimate things at their true value and to give the most effort to the things of greatest worth—the things that will endure.

This lesson is needed by those upon whom rests the responsibility of selecting a home. They should not allow themselves to be diverted from the highest aim. Let them remember that the home on earth is to be a symbol of and a preparation for the home in heaven. Life is a training school from which parents and children are to be graduated to the higher school in the mansions of God. As the location for a home is sought, let this purpose direct the choice. Do not be controlled by the desire for wealth, the dictates of fashion, or the customs of society. Consider what will tend most to simplicity, purity, health, and real worth.

Cities are becoming hotbeds of vice the world over. On every hand are the sights and sounds of evil. Everywhere are enticements to sensuality and dissipation. The tide of corruption and crime is continually swelling. Every day brings the record of violence—robberies, murders, suicides, and crimes unnamable.

Life in the cities is false and artificial. The intense passion for money getting, the whirl of excitement and pleasure seeking, the thirst for display, the luxury and extravagance, all are forces that, with the great masses of people, turn the mind from life's true purpose. They open the door to a thousand evils. Upon the youth they have almost irresistible power.

One of the most subtle and dangerous temptations that assail the children and youth in the cities is the love of pleasure. Holidays are numerous; sports events draw thousands, and the whirl of excitement and pleasure attracts them away from the sober duties of life. Money that should be saved for better uses is frittered away on amusements.

Through the working of monopolies and the results of labor unions and strikes, conditions of life in the city are constantly becoming more and more difficult. Serious troubles are before us, and for many families moving out of the cities will become a necessity.

The physical surroundings in the cities are often a peril to health. The constant likelihood of contact with disease, the prevalence of foul air, polluted water, impure food, the crowded, dark, unhealthful dwellings are some of the many evils to be met.

It was not God's purpose that people should be crowded into cities, huddled together in terraces and tenements. In the beginning He placed our first parents amidst the beautiful sights and sounds He desires us to rejoice in today. The more nearly we come into harmony with God's original plan, the better chance we will have to secure health of body and mind and soul.

Conditions for the Best Life

An expensive dwelling, elaborate furnishings, display, luxury, and ease do not furnish the conditions essential to a happy, useful life. Jesus came to this earth to accomplish the greatest work ever undertaken among us. He came as God's ambassador, to show us how to live so as to secure life's best results. What were the conditions chosen by the infinite Father for His Son? A secluded home in the Galilean hills; a household sustained by honest, self-respecting labor; a life of simplicity; daily conflict with difficulty and hardship; self-sacrifice, economy, and patient, gladsome service; the hour of study at His mother's side, with the open scroll of Scripture; the quiet of dawn or twilight in the green valley; the holy ministries of nature; the study of creation and providence; and the soul's communion with God— these were the conditions and opportunities of the early life of Jesus.

So with the great majority of the best and noblest people of all ages. Read the history of Abraham, Jacob, and Joseph, of Moses, David, and Elisha. Study the lives of men and women of later times who have most worthily filled positions of trust and responsibility, people whose influence has been most effective for the world's uplifting.

Many of these were reared in country homes. They knew little of luxury. They did not spend their youth in amusement. Many were forced to struggle with poverty and hardship. They early learned to work, and their active life in the open air gave vigor and elasticity to all their faculties. Forced to depend upon their own resources, they learned to combat difficulties and to surmount obstacles, and they gained courage and perseverance. They learned the lessons of self-reliance and self-control.

Sheltered to a great degree from evil associations, they were satisfied with natural pleasures and wholesome companionships. They were simple in their tastes and temperate in their habits. They were governed by principle, and they grew up pure and strong and true. When called to their lifework, they brought to it physical and mental power, buoyancy of spirit, ability to plan and execute, and steadfastness in resisting evil that made them a positive power for good in the world.

Better than any inheritance of wealth, give your children the gift of a healthy body, a sound mind, and a noble character. Understand what constitutes life's true success. Keep in view life's best things in your choice of a home.

Instead of dwelling where only the works of human beings can be seen, where the sights and sounds frequently suggest thoughts of evil, where turmoil and confusion bring weariness and disquietude, go where you can look upon the works of God. Find rest of spirit in the beauty and quietude and peace of nature. Let the eye rest on the green fields, the groves, and the hills. Look up to the blue sky, unobscured by the city's dust and smoke, and breathe the invigorating air of heaven. Go where, apart from the distractions and dissipations of city life, you can give your children your companionship, where you can teach them to learn of God through His works and train them for lives of integrity and usefulness.

Simplicity in Furnishing

Our artificial habits deprive us of many blessings and much enjoyment, and unfit us for living the most useful lives. Elaborate and expensive furnishings are a waste not only of money but of that which is a thousand-fold more precious. They bring into the home a heavy burden of care and labor and perplexity.

What are the conditions in many homes, even where resources are limited and the work of the household rests chiefly on the mother? The best rooms are furnished in a style beyond the means of the occupants and unsuited to their convenience and enjoyment. There are expensive carpets, elaborately carved and daintily upholstered furniture, and delicate drapery. Tables, mantels, and every other available space are crowded with ornaments, and the walls are covered with pictures, until the sight becomes wearying. And what an amount of work is required to keep all these in order and free from dust! This work, and the other artificial habits of the family in its conformity to fashion, demand of the housewife unending toil.

In many a home the wife and mother has no time to read, to keep herself well informed, no time to be a companion to her husband, no time to keep in touch with the developing minds of her children. There is no time or place for the precious Savior to be a close, dear companion. Little by little she sinks into a mere household drudge, her strength, time, and interest absorbed in the things that perish with the using. Too late she awakes to find herself almost a stranger in her own home. The precious opportunities to influence her dear ones for the higher life were left unimproved, and now have passed away forever.

Let homemakers resolve to live on a wiser plan. Let it be your first aim to make a pleasant home. Be sure to provide the facilities that will lighten labor and promote health and comfort. Plan for the entertainment of the guests whom Christ has told us to welcome and of whom He says, "Inasmuch as you did it to one of the least of these My brethren, you did it to Me." Matthew 25:40.

Furnish your home with things plain and simple, things that will bear handling, that can easily be kept clean, and that can be replaced without great expense. By exercising taste you can make a very simple home attractive and inviting, if love and contentment are there.

Beautiful Surroundings

God loves the beautiful. He has clothed the earth and the heavens with beauty, and with a Father's joy He watches the delight of His children in the things that He has made. He desires us to surround our homes with the beauty of natural things.

Nearly all dwellers in the country, however poor, could have around their homes a grassy lawn, a few shade trees, flowering shrubbery, or fragrant blossoms. And these things, far more than any artificial adorning, will minister to the happiness of the household. They will bring into the home life a softening, refining influence, strengthening the love of nature and drawing the members of the household nearer to one another and to God.

Chapter 31

The
Mother

To a great extent, what the parents are the children will be. The physical conditions of the parents, their dispositions and appetites, their mental and moral tendencies, are, to a greater or less degree, reproduced in their children.

The nobler the aims, the higher the mental and spiritual endowments, and the better developed the physical powers of the parents, the better will be the life equipment they give their children. In cultivating that which is best in themselves, parents are exerting an influence to mold society and to uplift future generations.

Fathers and mothers need to understand their responsibility. The world is full of snares for the feet of the young. Multitudes are attracted by a life of selfish and sensual pleasure. They cannot discern the hidden dangers or the fearful end to the path that seems to them the way of happiness. Through the indulgence of appetite and passion, their energies are wasted and millions are ruined for this world and for the world to come. Parents should remember that their children must encounter these temptations. Even before the birth of the child, the preparation should begin that will enable it to fight successfully the battle against evil.

Responsibility rests especially upon the mother. She, by whose life-blood the child is nourished and its physical frame built up, imparts to it also mental and spiritual influences that tend to shape both mind and character. It was Jochebed, the Hebrew mother, who, strong in faith, was "not afraid of the king's command." Hebrews 11:23. To her was born Moses, the deliverer of Israel. It was Hannah, the woman of prayer and self-sacrifice and heavenly inspiration, who gave birth to Samuel, the Heaven-instructed child, the incorruptible judge, the founder of Israel's sacred schools. It was Elizabeth, the kinswoman and kindred spirit of Mary of Nazareth, who was the mother of John, the Savior's herald.

Temperance and Self-Control

The carefulness with which the mother should guard her habits of life is taught in the Scriptures. When the Lord would raise up Samson as a deliverer for Israel, the angel of the Lord appeared to the mother, with special instruction concerning her habits, and also for the treatment of her child. "'Now drink no wine or similar drink, nor eat anything unclean,'" he said. Judges 13:13, 7.

Many parents look upon the effect of prenatal influences as a matter of little importance, but Heaven does not so regard it. The message sent by an angel of God, and twice given in the most solemn manner, shows it to be deserving of our most careful thought.

In the words spoken to the Hebrew mother, God speaks to all mothers in every age. "Let her be careful," the angel said; "All that I commanded her let her observe." The well-being of the child will be affected by the habits of the mother. Her appetites and passions are to be controlled by principle. There is something for her to shun, something for her to work against, if she fulfills God's purpose for her in giving her a child. If before the birth of her child she is self-indulgent, if she is selfish, impatient, and exacting, these traits will be reflected in the disposition of the child. Thus many children have received as a birthright almost unconquerable tendencies to evil.

But if the mother unswervingly adheres to right principles, if she is temperate and self-denying, if she is kind, gentle, and unselfish, she may give her child these same precious traits of character. Very explicit was the command prohibiting the use of wine by the mother. Every drop of strong drink taken by her to gratify appetite endangers the physical, mental, and moral health of her child, and is a direct sin against her Creator.

Many advisers urge that every wish of the mother be gratified; that if she desires any article of food, however harmful, she should freely indulge her appetite. Such advice is false and mischievous. In no case should the mother's physical needs be neglected. Two lives are depending upon her; her wishes should be tenderly regarded, her needs generously supplied. But at this time above all others she should avoid, in diet and in every other line, whatever would lessen physical or mental strength. By the command of God Himself she is placed under the most solemn obligation to exercise self-control.

Overwork

The strength of the mother should be tenderly cherished. Instead of spending her precious strength in exhausting labor, her care and burdens should be lessened. Often the husband and father is unacquainted with the physical laws that the well-being of his family requires him to understand. Absorbed in the struggle for a livelihood, or bent on acquiring wealth, he allows burdens to rest upon the wife and mother that overtax her strength at the most critical period. Feebleness and disease may result.

Many a husband and father might learn a helpful lesson from the carefulness of a faithful shepherd. Jacob, when urged to undertake a rapid and difficult journey, answered: "'The children are weak, and the flocks and herds which are nursing are with me. And if the men should drive them hard one day, all the flock will die. . . . I will lead on slowly at a pace which the livestock that go before me, and the children, are able to endure.'" Genesis 33:13, 14.

In life's toilsome way let the husband and father "lead on slowly," as the companion of his journey is able to endure. Amidst the world's eager rush for wealth and power, let him learn to slow down, to comfort and support the one who is called to walk by his side.

Cheerfulness

The mother should cultivate a cheerful, contented, happy disposition. Every effort in this direction will be abundantly repaid in both the physical well-being and the moral character of her children. A cheerful spirit will promote the happiness of her family and in a very great degree improve her own health.

Let the husband aid his wife by his sympathy and unfailing affection. If he wishes to keep her fresh and happy, so that she will be as sunshine in the home, let him help bear her burdens. His kindness and loving courtesy will be to her a precious encouragement, and the happiness he imparts will bring joy and peace to his own heart.

The husband and father who is morose, selfish, and overbearing is not only unhappy himself, he casts gloom upon all who live in his home. He will reap the result in seeing his wife dispirited and sickly, and his children marred with his own unlovely temper.

If the mother is deprived of the care and comforts she should have, if she is allowed to exhaust her strength through overwork or through anxiety and gloom, her children will be robbed of the strength, mental adaptability, and cheerful buoyancy they should inherit. It will be far better to make the mother's life bright and cheerful, to shield her from want, wearing labor, and depressing care, so that the children may inherit good constitutions and may battle their way through life with their own energetic strength.

Great is the honor and responsibility placed upon fathers and mothers, in that they are to stand in the place of God to their children. Their character, their daily life, their methods of training will interpret His words to the little ones. Their influence will win or repel the child's confidence in the Lord's assurances.

The Privilege of Parents in Child Training

Happy are the parents whose lives are a true reflection of the divine, so that the promises and commands of God awaken in their children gratitude and reverence. Happy are the parents whose tenderness, justice, and longsuffering reflect to the children the love and justice and longsuffering of God, parents who, by teaching their children to love and trust and obey them, are teaching them to love and trust and obey their Father in heaven. Parents who impart to their children such a gift have endowed them with a treasure more precious than the wealth of all the ages—a treasure as enduring as eternity.

In the children committed to her care, every mother has a sacred charge from God. "Take this son, this daughter," He says, "train it for Me; give it a character polished after the similitude of a palace, that it may shine in the courts of the Lord forever."

The mother's work often seems to her an unimportant service. Her work is rarely appreciated. Others know little of her many cares and burdens. Her days are occupied with a round of duties, all calling for patient effort, for self-control, for tact, wisdom, and self-sacrificing love, yet she cannot boast of what she has done as any great achievement. She has only kept things in the home running smoothly. Often weary and perplexed, she has tried to speak kindly to the children, to keep them busy and happy, and to guide their feet in the right path. She feels that she has accomplished nothing. But it is not so. Heavenly angels watch the care-worn mother, noting the burdens she carries day by day. Her name may not have been heard in the world, but it is written in the Lamb's book of life.

The Mother's Opportunity

There is a God above, and the light and glory from His throne rests upon the faithful mother as she tries to educate her children to resist the influence of evil. No other work can equal hers in importance. She has not, like the artist, to paint a form of beauty upon canvas, nor, like the sculptor, to chisel it from marble. She has not, like the author, to embody a noble thought in words of power, nor, like the musician, to express a beautiful sentiment in melody. It is hers, with the help of God, to develop in a human soul the likeness of the divine.

The mother who appreciates this will regard her opportunities as priceless. In her own character and by her methods of training, she will seek to present before her children the highest ideal. Earnestly, patiently, courageously, she will endeavor to improve her own abilities, that she may use properly the highest powers of the mind in training her children. Earnestly will she inquire at every step, "What has God said?" Diligently she will study His Word. She will keep her eyes fixed upon Christ, that her own daily experience, in the lowly round of care and duty, may be a true reflection of the one true Life.

C h a p t e r   32

The
Child

Not only the habits of the mother but the training of the child were included in the angel's instruction to Samson's Hebrew parents. It was not enough that the child who was to deliver Israel should have a good legacy at his birth; this was to be followed by careful training. From infancy he was to be trained to habits of strict temperance.

Similar instruction was given in regard to John the Baptist. Before the birth of the child, the message sent from heaven to the father was: "'You will have joy and gladness, and many will rejoice at his birth. For he will be great in the sight of the Lord, and shall drink neither wine nor strong drink. He will also be filled with the Holy Spirit.'" Luke 1:14, 15.

On heaven's record of noble men the Savior declared that no one was greater than John the Baptist. The work committed to him demanded not only physical energy and endurance but the highest qualities of mind and soul. So important was right physical training as a preparation for this work that the highest angel in heaven was sent with a message of instruction to the parents of the child.

The directions given concerning the Hebrew children teach us that nothing which affects the child's physical well-being is to be neglected. Nothing is unimportant. Every influence that affects the health of the body has its bearing upon mind and character.

Nothing is more important than the early training of children. The lessons learned, the habits formed during the years of infancy and childhood have more to do with the formation of the character and the direction of the life than have all the instruction and training of after years.

Parents need to consider this. They should understand the principles that underlie the care and training of children. They should be capable of rearing them in physical, mental, and moral health. Parents should study the laws of nature. They should become acquainted with the organism of the human body. They need to understand the functions of the various organs and their relation and dependence. They should study the relation of the mental to the physical powers and the conditions required for the healthy action of each. To assume the responsibilities of parenthood without such preparation is a sin.

Far too little thought is given to the causes underlying the mortality, the disease and degeneracy, that exist today even in the most civilized and favored lands. The human race is deteriorating. More than one third die in infancy.* Of those who reach manhood and womanhood, by far the greater number suffer from disease in some form, and but few reach the limit of human life.

Most of the evils that are bringing misery and ruin to the race might be prevented, and the power to deal with them rests to a great degree with parents. It is not a "mysterious providence" that removes little children by death. God does not want them to die. He gives them to the parents to be trained for usefulness here and for heaven hereafter. If fathers and mothers would do what they might to give their children a good inheritance, and then by right management endeavor to remedy any wrong conditions of their birth, what a change for the better the world might see!

The Care of Infants

The more quiet and simple the life of the child, the more favorable it will be for both physical and mental development. At all times the mother should endeavor to be quiet, calm, and self-possessed. Many infants are extremely susceptible to nervous excitement, and the mother's gentle, unhurried manner will have a soothing influence that will be of untold benefit to the child.

Babies require warmth, but a serious error often is committed in keeping them in overheated rooms, deprived to a great degree of fresh air. The practice of covering the infant's face while sleeping is harmful, since it prevents free respiration.

The baby should be kept free from every influence that would tend to weaken or poison the system. The most scrupulous care should be taken to have everything about it sweet and clean. While it may be necessary to protect the little ones from sudden or too great changes of temperature, care should be taken that, sleeping or waking, day or night, they breathe a pure, invigorating atmosphere. In the preparation of the baby's wardrobe, convenience, comfort, and health should take priority over fashion or a desire to excite admiration. The mother should not spend time in embroidery and fancywork to make the

---

*The statement concerning infant mortality was correct at the time it was written in 1905. However, modern medicine and proper child care have greatly reduced the mortality rate in infancy and childhood in many countries.—Publisher.

little garments beautiful, thus taxing herself with unnecessary work at the expense of her own health and the health of her child. She should not do sewing that severely taxes eyes and nerves at a time when she needs much rest and pleasant exercise. She should realize her obligation to cherish her strength, that she may be able to meet the demands that will be made upon her.

If the dress of the child combines warmth, protection, and comfort, one of the chief causes of irritation and restlessness will be removed. The little one will have better health, and the mother will not find the care of the child so heavy a tax upon her strength and time.

Tight bands or waists hinder the action of the heart and lungs, and should be avoided. No part of the body should at any time be made uncomfortable by clothing that compresses any organ or restricts its freedom of movement. The clothing of all children should be loose enough to admit of the freest and fullest respiration, and so arranged that the shoulders will support its weight.

In some countries the custom of leaving bare the shoulders and limbs of little children still prevails. This custom cannot be too severely condemned. The limbs, being remote from the center of circulation, demand greater protection than other parts of the body. The arteries that convey the blood to the extremities are large, providing for a sufficient quantity of blood to afford warmth and nutrition. But when the limbs are left unprotected or are insufficiently clad, the arteries and veins become contracted, the sensitive portions of the body are chilled, and the circulation of the blood is hindered.

In growing children all the forces of nature need every advantage to enable them to perfect the physical frame. If the arms and legs are insufficiently protected, children, and especially girls, are not allowed to go out of doors unless the weather is mild. So they are kept in for fear of the cold. But if children are well clothed, it will benefit them to exercise freely in the open air, summer or winter.

Mothers who desire their boys and girls to possess the vigor of health should dress them properly and encourage them in all reasonable weather to be much in the open air. It may require effort to ignore custom and to dress and educate the children with reference to health, but the result will amply repay the effort.

The Child's Diet

The best food for the infant is breast milk, the food that nature provides. Of this it should not be needlessly deprived. It is a heartless thing for a mother, for the sake of convenience or social enjoyment, to free herself from the tender office of nursing her little one.

The mother who permits her child to be nourished by another should consider well what the result may be. To a greater or less degree the nurse imparts her own temper and temperament to the nursing child.

The importance of training children to right habits of diet can hardly be overestimated. The little ones need to learn that they eat to live, not live to eat. The training should begin with the infant in its mother's arms. The child should be given food only at regular intervals, and less frequently as it grows older. It should not be given sweets, or the food of older persons, which it is unable to digest. Care and regularity in the feeding of infants will not only promote health, and thus tend to make them quiet and sweet-tempered, it will lay the foundation of habits that will be a blessing to them in after years.

As children emerge from babyhood, great care should still be taken in educating their tastes and appetite. Often they are permitted to eat what they choose and when they choose, without reference to health. The pains and money so often lavished upon unwholesome delicacies lead the young to think that the highest object in life, and that which yields the greatest amount of happiness, is to be able to indulge the appetite. The result of this training is gluttony, then comes sickness, which is usually followed by dosing with poisonous drugs.

Parents should train the appetites of their children and not permit the use of unwholesome foods. But in the effort to regulate the diet, they should be careful not to err in requiring children to eat that which is distasteful, or to eat more than is needed. Children have rights, they have preferences, and when these preferences are reasonable they should be respected.

Regularity in eating should be carefully observed. Nothing should be eaten between meals—no confectionery, nuts, fruits, or food of any kind. Irregularities in eating destroy the healthful tone of the digestive organs, to the detriment of health and cheerfulness. And when the children come to the table, they do not relish wholesome food; their appetites crave that which is hurtful for them.

Mothers who gratify the desires of their children at the expense of health and happy tempers are sowing seeds of evil that will spring up and bear fruit. Self-indulgence grows with the growth of the little ones, and both mental and physical vigor are sacrificed. Mothers who do this work reap with bitterness the seed they have sown. They see their children grow up unfitted in mind and character to act a noble and useful part in society or in the home. The spiritual as well as the mental and physical powers suffer under the influence of unhealthful food. The conscience becomes insensitive, and the susceptibility to good impressions is impaired.

While the children should be taught to control the appetite and to eat with reference to health, make it plain that they are denying themselves only that which would do them harm. They give up hurtful things for something better. Let the table be made inviting and attractive, as it is supplied with the good things that God has so bountifully bestowed. Make mealtime a cheerful, happy time. As we enjoy the gifts of God, let us respond by grateful praise to the Giver.

The Care of Children in Sickness

In many cases the sickness of children can be traced to errors in management. Irregularities in eating, insufficient clothing when the weather is chilly, lack of vigorous exercise to keep the blood in healthy circulation, or lack of abundance of air for its purification may be the cause of the trouble. Let the parents study to find the causes of the sickness and then remedy the wrong conditions as soon as possible.

All parents have it in their power to learn much concerning the care and prevention, and even the treatment, of disease. The mother especially ought to know what to do in common cases of illness in her family. She should know how to minister to her sick child. Her love and insight should fit her to perform services for it that could not so well be trusted to a stranger's hand.

The Study of Physiology

Parents should early seek to interest their children in the study of the human body and should teach them the simpler principles on which the body's organs work. Teach them how best to preserve the physical, mental, and spiritual powers, and how to use their gifts so that their lives may bring blessing to one another and honor to God. This knowledge is invaluable to the young. An education in the things that concern life and health is more important to them than a knowledge of many of the sciences taught in the schools.

Parents should live more for their children, and less for society. Study health subjects, and put your knowledge to a practical use. Teach your children to reason from cause to effect. Teach them that if they desire health and happiness, they must obey the laws of nature. Though you may not see as rapid improvement as you desire, do not be discouraged, but patiently and perseveringly continue your work.

From babyhood onward, teach your children to practice self-denial and self-control. Teach them to enjoy the beauties of nature and in useful activities to exercise systematically all the powers of body and mind. Bring them up to have sound constitutions and good morals, to have sunny dispositions and sweet tempers. Impress upon their tender minds the truth that God does not design that we should live merely for present gratification, but for our ultimate good. Teach them that to yield to temptation is weak and wicked; to resist, strong and noble. These lessons will be as seed sown in good soil, and they will bear fruit that will make your hearts glad.

Above all else, let parents surround their children with an atmosphere of cheerfulness, courtesy, and love. A home where love dwells, and where it is expressed in looks, in words, and in acts, is a place where angels delight to manifest their presence.

Parents, let the sunshine of love, cheerfulness, and happy contentment enter your own hearts, and let its sweet, cheering influence pervade your home. Manifest a kindly, forbearing spirit, and encourage the same in your children, cultivating all the graces that will brighten the home life. The atmosphere thus created will be to the children what air and sunshine are to the vegetable world, promoting health and vigor of mind and body.

C h a p t e r   33

Home
Influences

Home should be to children the most attractive place in the world, and the mother's presence should be its greatest attraction. Children have sensitive, loving natures. They are easily pleased and easily made unhappy. By gentle discipline, in loving words and acts, mothers may bind their children to their hearts.

Young children love companionship and can seldom enjoy themselves alone. They yearn for sympathy and tenderness. They think that whatever they enjoy will please mother also, and it is natural for them to go to her with their little joys and sorrows. The mother should not wound their sensitive hearts by treating with indifference matters that, though trifling to her, are of great importance to them. Her sympathy and approval are precious. An approving glance, a word of encouragement or commendation will be like sunshine in their hearts, often making their whole day happy.

Instead of sending her children from her, that she may not be annoyed by their noise or troubled by their little wants, let the mother plan amusement or light work to employ the active hands and minds.

By entering into their feelings and directing their amusements and employments, the mother will gain the confidence of her children. This will enable her more effectually to correct wrong habits or check the manifestations of selfishness or passion. A word of caution or reproof spoken at the right time will be of great value. By patient, watchful love, she can turn the minds of the children in the right direction, cultivating in them beautiful and attractive traits of character.

Mothers should guard against training their children to be dependent and self-absorbed. Never lead them to think that they are the center and that everything must revolve around them. Some parents give much time and attention to amusing their children, but children should be trained to amuse themselves, to exercise their own ingenuity and skill. Thus they will learn to be content with very simple pleasures. They should be taught to bear bravely their disappointments and trials. Instead of calling attention to every trifling pain or hurt, divert their minds; teach them to pass lightly over little annoyances or discomforts. Study to suggest ways by which the children may learn to be thoughtful of others.

But do not neglect the children. Burdened with many cares, mothers sometimes feel that they cannot take time patiently to instruct their little ones and give them love and sympathy. They should remember that if the children do not find in their parents and in their home that which will satisfy their need for sympathy and companionship, they will look to other sources, where both mind and character may be endangered.

For lack of time and thought, many a mother refuses her children some innocent pleasure, while her busy fingers and weary eyes are diligently engaged in work designed only for adornment, something that likely will serve only to encourage vanity and extravagance in their young hearts. As the children approach manhood and womanhood, these lessons bear fruit in pride and moral worthlessness. The mother grieves over her children's faults but does not realize that the harvest she is reaping is from seed that she herself planted.

Some mothers are not uniform in the treatment of their children. At times they indulge them to their injury; at other times they refuse some innocent gratification that would make the childish heart very happy. In this they do not imitate Christ. He loved the children. He comprehended their feelings and sympathized with them in their pleasures and their trials.

The Father's Responsibility

The husband and father is the head of the household. The wife looks to him for love and sympathy, and for aid in training the children. This is right; the children are his as well as hers, and he is equally interested in their welfare. The children look to their father for support and guidance. He needs to have a right conception of life and of the influences and associations that should surround his family. Above all, he should be controlled by the love and fear of God and by the teaching of His Word, that he may guide the feet of his children in the right way.

The father is the lawmaker of the household, and, like Abraham, he should make the law of God the rule of his home. God said of Abraham, "I know him, that he will command his children and his household." Genesis 18:19, KJV. There would be no sinful neglect to restrain evil, no weak, unwise, indulgent favoritism, no yielding of his conviction of duty to the claims of mistaken affection. Abraham would not only give right instruction, he would maintain the authority of just and righteous laws. God has given rules for our guidance. Children should not be left to wander away from the safe path marked out in God's Word into ways leading to danger, which are open on every side. Kindly but firmly, with persevering, prayerful effort, their wrong desires should be restrained, their evil inclinations denied.

The father should enforce in his family the sterner virtues—energy, integrity, honesty, patience, courage, diligence, and practical usefulness. And what he requires of his children he himself should practice, illustrating these virtues in his own life.

But, fathers, do not discourage your children. Combine affection with authority, kindness and sympathy with firm restraint. Give some of your leisure hours to your children; become acquainted with them; associate with them in their work and in their sports, and win their confidence. Cultivate friendship with them, especially with your sons. In this way you will be a strong influence for good.

The father should do his part toward making home happy. Whatever his cares and business perplexities, they should not be permitted to affect his family; he should enter his home with smiles and pleasant words.

In a sense the father is the priest of the household, laying upon the family altar the morning and evening sacrifice. But the wife and children should unite in prayer and join in the song of praise. In the morning before he leaves home for his daily work, the father should gather his children about him and, bowing before God, commit them to the care of the Father in heaven. When the cares of the day are past, let the family unite in grateful prayer and a song of praise, acknowledging divine care during the day.

Fathers and mothers, however pressing your business, do not fail to gather your family together to worship God. Ask for the guardianship of holy angels in your home. Remember that your dear ones are exposed to temptations. Daily annoyances beset the path of young and old. Those who would live patient, loving, cheerful lives must pray. Only by receiving constant help from God can we gain the victory over self.

Happiness and Love Are Important

Home should be a place of cheerfulness, courtesy, and love. Where these graces prevail, there will be happiness and peace. Troubles may invade, but these are the lot of humanity. Let patience, gratitude, and love keep sunshine in the heart though the day may be ever so cloudy. In such homes angels of God abide.

Let the husband and wife study each other's happiness, never failing in the small courtesies and kindly acts that cheer and brighten the life. Perfect confidence should exist between husband and wife. Together they should consider their responsibilities. Together they should work for the highest good of their children. Never should they in the presence of the children criticize each other's plans or question each other's judgment. Let the wife be careful not to make the husband's work for the children more difficult. Let the husband hold up the hands of his wife, giving her wise counsel and loving encouragement.

No barrier of coldness and reserve should be allowed to arise between parents and children. Let parents become acquainted with their children, seeking to understand their tastes and dispositions, entering into their feelings, and drawing out what is in their hearts.

Parents, show your children that you love them and will do all in your power to make them happy. If you do this, your necessary restrictions will have far greater weight in their young minds. Rule your children with tenderness and compassion, remembering that "'their angels always see the face of My Father who is in heaven.'" Matthew 18:10. If you want the angels to do for your children the work given them of God, cooperate with them by doing your part.

Brought up under the wise and loving guidance of a true home, children will have no desire to wander away in search of pleasure and companionship. Evil will not attract them. The spirit that prevails in the home will mold their characters; they will form habits and principles that will be a strong defense against temptation when they leave the home shelter and take their place in the world.

Children as well as parents have important duties in the home. They should be taught that they are a part of the home firm. They are fed and clothed and loved and cared for, and they should respond to these many mercies by carrying their share of the home burdens and bringing all the happiness possible into the family of which they are members.

Children are sometimes tempted to chafe under restraint, but when they become adults they will bless their parents for the faithful care and strict watchfulness that guarded and guided them in their years of inexperience.

True Education
a Missionary Training

True education is missionary training. Every son and daughter of God is called to be a missionary. We are called to serve God and one another. To fit us for this service should be the object of our education.

This object should ever be kept in view by Christian parents and teachers. We know not in what line our children may serve. They may spend their lives within the circle of the home. They may engage in life's common vocations or go as teachers of the gospel to heathen lands. But all are alike called to be missionaries for God, ministers of mercy to the world.

The children and youth, with their fresh talent, energy, courage, and quick susceptibilities, are loved of God, and He desires to bring them into harmony with divine agencies. They are to obtain an education that will help them stand by the side of Christ in unselfish service.

Of all His children to the close of time, no less than of the first disciples, Christ said, "'As You sent Me into the world, I also have sent them into the world'" (John 17:18), to be representatives of God, to reveal His Spirit, to manifest His character, to do His work.

Our children stand, as it were, at the parting of the ways. On every hand the world's enticements to self-seeking and self-indulgence call them away from the path that leads to the Holy City. Whether their lives shall be a blessing or a curse depends upon the choices they make. Overflowing with energy, eager to test their untried capabilities, they must find some outlet for their superabounding life. Active they will be for good or for evil.

God's Word does not repress activity, but guides it aright. God does not tell the youth to be less aspiring. The elements of character that make a person truly successful and honored by peers—the irrepressible desire for some greater good, the indomitable will, the strenuous application, the untiring perseverance—are not to be discouraged. By the grace of God they are to be directed to the attainment of objects as much higher than selfish and worldly interests as the heavens are higher than the earth.

It rests with us as parents and as Christians to give our children right direction. They are to be carefully, wisely, tenderly guided into paths of Christlike ministry. We are under sacred covenant with God to rear our children for His service. Our first duty is to surround them with such influences as shall lead them to choose a life of service, and to give them the training needed.

"God so loved . . . that He gave," "gave His only begotten Son," that we "should not perish but have everlasting life." "Christ . . . has loved us and given Himself for us." If we love, we shall give. "Not . . . to be served, but to serve" is the great lesson that we are to learn and teach. John 3:16; Ephesians 5:2; Matthew 20:28.

Impress the youth with the thought that they are not their own. They belong to Christ. They are the purchase of His blood, the claim of His love. They live because He keeps them by His power. Their time, their strength, their capabilities are His, to be developed, to be trained, to be used for Him.

Next to the angelic beings, the human family, formed in the image of God, are the noblest of His created works. God desires them to become all that He has made it possible for them to be, and to do their very best with the powers He has given them.

Life is mysterious and sacred. It is the manifestation of God Himself, the Source of all life. Precious are its opportunities. Earnestly should they be improved. Once lost, they are gone forever.

Before us God places eternity, with its solemn realities, and gives us a grasp on immortal, imperishable themes. He presents valuable, ennobling truth, that we may advance in a safe and sure path, in pursuit of an object worthy of the earnest engagement of all our capabilities.

God looks into the tiny seed that He Himself has formed, and sees wrapped within it the beautiful flower, the shrub, or the lofty, wide-spreading tree. So also He sees the possibilities in every human being. We are here for a purpose. God has given us His plan for our life, and He wants us to reach the highest standard of development.

He desires that we shall constantly be growing in holiness, in happiness, in usefulness. All have capabilities that they must be taught to regard as sacred endowments, to appreciate as the Lord's gifts, and rightly to employ. He desires the youth to cultivate every power of their being and to bring every faculty into active exercise. He desires them to enjoy all that is useful and precious in this life, to be good and to do good, laying up a heavenly treasure for the future life.

It should be their ambition to excel in all things that are unselfish, high, and noble. Let them look to Christ as their Pattern. They are to cherish the holy ambition that He revealed in His life—an ambition to make the world better for their having lived in it. This is the work to which they are called.

A Broad Foundation

The highest of all sciences is the science of soul saving. The greatest work to which human beings can aspire is the work of winning men and women from sin to holiness. For the accomplishment of this work, a broad foundation must be laid. A comprehensive education is needed—an education that will demand from parents and teachers such thought and effort as mere instruction in the sciences does not require. Something more is called for than the culture of the intellect. Education is not complete unless the body, mind, and heart are equally educated. The character must receive proper discipline for its fullest and highest development. All the faculties of mind and body are to be developed and rightly trained. It is a duty to cultivate and exercise every power that will render us more efficient workers for God.

True education includes the whole being. It teaches the right use of one's self. It enables us to make the best use of brain, bone, and muscle, of body, mind, and heart. The faculties of the mind, as the higher powers, are to rule the kingdom of the body. The natural appetites and passions are to be brought under the control of the conscience and the spiritual affections. Christ stands at the head of humanity, and it is His purpose to lead us, in His service, into high and holy paths of purity. By the wondrous working of His grace we are to be made complete in Him.

Jesus received His education in the home. His mother was His first human teacher. From her lips and from the scrolls of the prophets, He learned of heavenly things. He lived in a peasant's home, faithfully and cheerfully acting His part in bearing the household burdens. He who had been the commander of heaven was a willing servant, a loving, obedient son. He learned a trade and with His own hands worked in the carpenter's shop with Joseph. In the garb of a common laborer He walked the streets of the little town, going to and returning from His humble work.

The people of that age estimated the value of things by outward show. As religion had declined in power, it had increased in pomp. The educators of the time sought to command respect by display and ostentation. To all this the life of Jesus presented a marked contrast. His life demonstrated the worthlessness of those things widely regarded as life's great essentials. He did not attend the schools of His time, with their magnifying of things small and their belittling of things great. His education was gained from Heaven-appointed sources—useful work, study of the Scriptures, nature, and the experiences of life. These lesson books of God are full of instruction to all who bring to them the willing hand, the seeing eye, and the understanding heart.

"The Child grew and became strong in spirit, filled with wisdom; and the grace of God was upon Him." Luke 2:40.

Thus prepared, He went forth to His mission, in every moment of His contact with men and women exerting upon them an influence to bless, a power to transform, such as the world had never witnessed.

The home is the child's first school, and it is here that the foundation should be laid for a life of service. Its principles are to be taught not merely in theory; they are to shape the whole life training.

Very early the lesson of helpfulness should be taught to children. As soon as strength and reasoning power are sufficiently developed, children should be given duties to perform in the home. They should be encouraged to try helping father and mother, to deny and to control themselves, to put others' happiness and convenience before their own, to watch for opportunities to cheer and assist brothers and sisters and playmates, and to show kindness to the aged, the sick, and the unfortunate. The more fully the spirit of true ministry pervades the home, the more fully it will be developed in the lives of the children. They will learn to find joy in service and sacrifice for the good of others.

The Work of the School

The home training should be supplemented by the work of the school. The development of the whole being, physical, mental, and spiritual, and the teaching of service and sacrifice, should be kept constantly in view.

Above any other agency, service for Christ's sake in the little things of everyday experience has power to mold the character and direct the life into lines of unselfish ministry. To awaken this spirit, to encourage and rightly to direct it, is the parents' and the teachers' work. No more important work could be committed to them. The spirit of ministry is the spirit of heaven, and angels will cooperate with every effort to develop and encourage it.

Such an education must be based upon the Word of God. Here only are its principles given in their fullness. The Bible should be made the foundation of study and of teaching. The essential knowledge is a knowledge of God and of Him whom He has sent.

Every child and every youth should have a knowledge of himself or herself. Both boys and girls should understand the physical habitation that God has given them and the laws by which it is kept in health. All should be thoroughly grounded in the common branches of education. And they should have industrial training that will make them men and women of practical ability, fitted for the duties of everyday life. To this should be added training and practical experience in various lines of missionary effort.

Learning by Imparting

Let the youth advance as fast and as far as they can in acquiring knowledge. Their field of study should be as broad as their powers can compass. And, as they learn, they should impart their knowledge. Thus their minds will acquire discipline and power. It is the use they make of knowledge that determines the value of their education. To spend a long time in study, with no effort to impart what is gained, often proves a hindrance rather than a help to real development.

In both the home and the school, students should learn how to study and how to impart the knowledge gained. Whatever their calling, they are to be both learners and teachers as long as life shall last. Thus they may advance continually, making God their trust, clinging to Him who is infinite in wisdom, who can reveal the secrets hidden for ages, who can solve the most difficult problems for minds that believe in Him.

God's Word places great emphasis upon the influence of association, even upon mature people. How much greater is its power on the developing minds and characters of children and youth! The company they keep, the principles they adopt, the habits they form, will decide the question of their usefulness here and of their future, eternal interest.

It is a terrible fact, and one that should make the hearts of parents tremble, that in many schools and colleges to which the youth are sent for mental culture and discipline, influences prevail that misshape the character, divert the mind from life's true aims, and debase the morals. Through contact with irreligious, pleasure loving, and corrupt associates, many youth lose the simplicity and purity, the faith in God, and the spirit of self-sacrifice that Christian fathers and mothers have cherished and guarded by careful instruction and earnest prayer.

Many who enter school with the purpose of fitting themselves for some line of unselfish ministry become absorbed in secular studies. Their ambition is aroused to win distinction in scholarship and to gain position and honor in the world. They lose sight of the purpose for which they entered school, and their life is given up to selfish and worldly pursuits. Often habits are formed that ruin the life both for this world and for the world to come.

As a rule, men and women who have broad ideas, unselfish purposes, noble aspirations, are those in whom these characteristics were developed by their associations in early years. In all His dealings with Israel, God urged upon them the importance of guarding the associations of their children. All the arrangements of civil, religious, and social life were made with a view to preserving the children from harmful companionship and making them, from their earliest years, familiar with the precepts and principles of the law of God. The object lesson given at the birth of the nation was of a nature to impress deeply all hearts.

Before the last terrible judgment came upon the Egyptians in the death of the first-born, God commanded His people to gather their children into their own homes. The doorpost of every house was marked with blood, and all were to abide within the protection assured by this token. So today parents who love and fear God are to keep their children under "the bond of the covenant"—within the protection of those sacred influences made possible through Christ's redeeming blood.

Of His disciples Christ said, "'I have given them Your word; and . . . they are not of the world, just as I am not of the world.'" John 17:14.

"Do not be conformed to this world," God bids us, "but be transformed by the renewing of your mind." Romans 12:2.

"Do not be unequally yoked together with unbelievers. For what fellowship has righteousness with lawlessness? And what communion has light with darkness? . . . And what agreement has the temple of God with idols? For you are the temple of the living God. As God has said: 'I will dwell in them and walk among them. I will be their God, and they shall be My people.' Therefore

'Come out from among them and be separate, . . .
Do not touch what is unclean,
And I will receive you.'
'I will be a Father to you,
And you shall be My sons and daughters,
Says the Lord Almighty.'"
2 Corinthians 6:14-18.

"Gather the children." "Make them know the statutes of God, and his laws." Joel 2:16; Exodus 18:16, KJV.

"'Put My name on the children of Israel, and I will bless them.'" Numbers 6:27. "'All peoples of the earth shall see that you are called by the name of the Lord.'" Deuteronomy 28:10.

"The remnant of Jacob shall be in the midst of many peoples,
Like dew from the Lord,
Like showers on the grass,
That tarry for no man
Nor wait for the sons of men."
Micah 5:7.

We are numbered with Israel. All the instruction given to the Israelites of old concerning the education and training of their children, all the promises of blessing through obedience, are for us. God's word to us is, "I will bless you . . . and you shall be a blessing." Genesis 12:2.

Of the first disciples and of all who should believe on Him through their word Christ said, "'The glory which You gave Me I have given them, that they may be one just as We are one; I in them, and You in Me; that they may be made perfect in one, and that the world may know that You have sent Me, and have loved them as You have loved Me.'" John 17:22, 23.

Wonderful, wonderful words, almost beyond the grasp of faith! The Creator of all worlds loves those who give themselves to His service, even as He loves His Son. Even here and now His gracious favor is bestowed upon us to this marvelous extent. He has given us the Light and Majesty of heaven, and with Him He has bestowed all the heavenly treasure. Much as He has promised us rich rewards in the life to come, so also He bestows princely gifts in this life. As subjects of His grace, He desires us to enjoy everything that will ennoble, expand, and elevate our characters. He is waiting to inspire the youth with power from above, that they may stand under the blood-stained banner of Christ, to work as He worked, to lead souls into safe paths, to plant the feet of many upon the Rock of Ages.

All who are seeking to work in harmony with God's plan of education will have His sustaining grace, His continual presence, His keeping power. To everyone He says:

"'Be strong and of good courage; do not be afraid, nor be dismayed, for the Lord your God is with you.'" "'I will not leave you nor forsake you.'" Joshua 1:9, 5.

> "'As the rain comes down, and the snow from heaven,
> And do not return there,
> But water the earth, and make it bring forth and bud,
> That it may give seed to the sower and bread to the eater,
> So shall My word be that goes forth from My mouth;
> It shall not return to Me void,
> But it shall accomplish what I please,
> And it shall prosper in the thing for which I sent it.
> For you shall go out with joy,
> And be led out with peace;
> The mountains and the hills shall break forth
>   into singing before you.
> And all the trees of the field shall clap their hands.
> Instead of the thorn shall come up the cypress tree,
> And instead of the brier shall come up the myrtle tree;
> And it shall be to the Lord for a name,
> For an everlasting sign that shall not be cut off.'"
> Isaiah 55:10-13.

Throughout the world, society is in disorder, and a thorough transformation is needed. The education given to the youth is to mold the whole social fabric.

"They shall rebuild the old ruins,
They shall raise up the former desolations,
And they shall repair the ruined cities,
The desolations of many generations."
People shall call them "the Servants of our God. . . .
Everlasting joy shall be theirs.
'For I, the Lord, love justice; . . .
I will direct their work in truth,
And will make with them an everlasting covenant.
Their descendants shall be known among the Gentiles,
And their offspring among the people.
All who see them shall acknowledge them,
That they are the posterity whom the Lord has blessed.' . . .
For as the earth brings forth its bud,
As the garden causes the things that are sown in it to spring forth,
So the Lord God will cause righteousness and praise to spring forth
    before all the nations."

                                       Isaiah 61:4, 6-8, 9, 11.

The Essential Knowledge

A True Knowledge of God

Like our Savior, we are in this world to do service for God. We are here to become like God in character, and by a life of service to reveal Him to the world. In order to be co-workers with God, in order to become like Him and to reveal His character, we must know Him aright. We must know Him as He reveals Himself.

A knowledge of God is the foundation of all true education and of all true service. It is the only real safeguard against temptation. This alone can make us like God in character.

This is the knowledge needed by all who are working to uplift others. Transformation of character, purity of life, efficiency in service, adherence to correct principles, all depend upon a right knowledge of God. This knowledge is the essential preparation both for this life and for the life to come.

"The knowledge of the Holy One is understanding." Proverbs 9:10. Through a knowledge of Him are given unto us "all things that pertain to life and godliness." 2 Peter 1:3.

"'This is eternal life,'" said Jesus, "'that they may know You, the only true God, and Jesus Christ whom You have sent.'" John 17:3.

"Thus says the Lord:
'Let not the wise man glory in his wisdom,
Let not the mighty man glory in his might,
Nor let the rich man glory in his riches;

But let him who glories glory in this,
That he understands and knows Me,
That I am the Lord, exercising lovingkindness,
      judgment, and righteousness in the earth.
For in these I delight,' says the Lord."
                              Jeremiah 9:23, 24.

We need to study the revelations of Himself that God has given.

"'Now acquaint yourself with Him,
And be at peace;
Thereby good will come to you.
Receive, please, instruction from His mouth,
And lay up His words in your heart' ". . . .

" 'Yes, the Almighty will be your gold
And your precious silver;
For then you will have your delight in the Almighty,
And lift up your face to God.
You will make your prayer to Him,
He will hear you,
And you will pay your vows.
You will also declare a thing,
And it will be established for you;
So light will shine on your ways.
When they cast you down, and you say,
      "Exaltation will come!"
Then He will save the humble person.'"
                              Job 22:21-29.

"Since the creation of the world His invisible attributes are clearly seen, being understood by the things that are made, even His eternal power and Godhead." Romans 1:20. The things of nature that we now see give us but a faint conception of Eden's glory. Sin has marred earth's beauty. On all things may be seen traces of the work of evil. Yet much that is beautiful remains. Nature testifies that One infinite in power, great in goodness, mercy, and love, created the earth and filled it with life and gladness. Even in their blighted state, all things reveal the handiwork of the great Master Artist. Wherever we turn, we may hear the voice of God and see evidences of His goodness.

From the solemn roll of the deep-toned thunder and the ocean's ceaseless roar to the glad songs that make the forests vocal with melody, nature's ten thousand voices speak His praise. In earth and sea and sky, with their marvelous tint and color, varying in gorgeous contrast or blended in harmony, we see His glory. The everlasting hills tell us of His power. The trees that wave their green banners in the sunlight and the flowers in their delicate beauty point to their Creator. The living green that carpets the brown earth tells of God's care for the humblest of His creatures. The caves of the sea and the depths of the earth reveal His treasures. He who placed the pearls in the ocean and the amethyst and chrysolite among the rocks is a lover of the beautiful. The sun rising in the heavens is a representative of Him who is the life and light of all that He has made. All the brightness and beauty that adorn the earth and light up the heavens speak of God. All things tell of His tender, fatherly care and of His desire to make His children happy.

"His glory covered the heavens."
"The earth is full of Your possessions."

"Day unto day utters speech,
And night unto night reveals knowledge.
There is no speech nor language
Where their voice is not heard.
Their line has gone out through all the earth,
And their words to the end of the world."
Habakkuk 3:3; Psalm 104:24; 19:2-4.

The mighty power that works through nature and sustains all things is not, as some scientists represent, merely an all-pervading principle, an actuating energy. God is a Spirit, yet He is a personal Being, for so He has revealed Himself.

"The Lord is the true God,
He is the living God and the everlasting King. . . .
'The gods that have not made the heavens and the earth
   shall perish from the earth and from under these heavens.' "

"The Portion of Jacob is not like them,
For He is the Maker of all things."

"He has made the earth by His power,
He has established the world by His wisdom,
And has stretched out the heavens at His discretion."
Jeremiah 10:10, 11, 16, 12.

Nature Is Not God

God's handiwork in nature is not God Himself in nature. The things of nature are an expression of God's character and power, but we are not to regard nature as God. The artistic skill of human beings produces very beautiful workmanship, things that delight the eye. These things reveal to us something of the thought of the designer, but the thing made is not the maker. It is not the work, but the workman, that is counted worthy of honor. So, while nature is an expression of God's thought, God, not nature, is to be exalted.

> "Let us worship and bow down;
> Let us kneel before the Lord our Maker."
> "In His hand are the deep places of the earth;
> The heights of the hills are His also.
> The sea is His, for He made it;
> And His hands formed the dry land."
>
> Psalm 95:6, 4, 5.

> "He made the Pleiades and Orion;
> He turns the shadow of death into morning
> And makes the day dark as night."
> "He who forms mountains, and creates the wind,
> Who declares to man what His thought is,"
> "He who builds His layers in the sky,
> And has founded His strata in the earth;
> Who calls for the waters of the sea,
> And pours them out on the face of the earth—
> The Lord is His name."
>
> Amos 5:8; 4:13; 9:6.

The Creation of the Earth

The work of creation cannot be explained by science. What science is there that can explain the mystery of life?

"By faith we understand that the worlds were framed by the word of God, so that the things which are seen were not made of things which are visible." Hebrews 11:3.

> " "I form the light and create darkness, . . .
> I, the Lord, do all these things." . . .
> I have made the earth,
> And created man on it.
> I—My hands—stretched out the heavens,
> And all their host I have commanded.' "
> " 'When I call to them, they stand up together.' "
>
> Isaiah 45:7, 12; 48:13.

In the creation of the earth, God was not indebted to preexisting matter. "He spoke, and it was . . . ; He commanded, and it stood fast." Psalm 33:9. All things, material or spiritual, stood up before the Lord God at His voice and were created for His own purpose. The heavens and all the host of them, the earth and everything in it, came into existence by the breath of His mouth.

In the creation of man was manifest the agency of a personal God. When God had made man in His image, the human form was perfect in all its arrangements, but it was without life. Then a personal, self-existing God breathed into that form the breath of life, and man became a living, intelligent being. All parts of the human organism were set in action. The heart, the arteries, the veins, the tongue, the hands, the feet, the senses, the faculties of the mind, all began their work, and all were placed under law. Man became a living soul. Through Christ the Word, a personal God created man and endowed him with intelligence and power.

Our substance was not hid from Him when we were made in secret; His eyes saw our substance, yet being imperfect, and in His book all our members were written when as yet there were none of them. (See Psalm 139:15, 16.)

Above all lower orders of life, God designed that human beings, the crowning work of His creation, should express His thought and reveal His glory. But humans are not to exalt themselves as God.

"Make a joyful shout to the Lord. . . .
Serve the Lord with gladness;
Come before His presence with singing.
Know that the Lord, He is God;
It is He who has made us, and not we ourselves;
We are His people and the sheep of His pasture.
Enter into His gates with thanksgiving,
And into His courts with praise.
Be thankful to Him, and bless His name."

"Exalt the Lord our God,
And worship at His holy hill;
For the Lord our God is holy."
                    Psalm 100:1-4; 99:9.

God is constantly employed in upholding and using as His servants the things that He has made. He works through the laws of nature, using them as His instruments. They are not self-acting. Nature in her work testifies of the intelligent presence and active agency of a Being who moves in all things according to His will.

"Forever, O Lord,
Your word is settled in heaven.
Your faithfulness endures to all generations;
You established the earth, and it abides.
They continue this day according to Your ordinances,
For all are Your servants."

"Whatever the Lord pleases He does,
In heaven and in earth,
In the seas and in all deep places."

"He commanded and they were created.
He also established them forever and ever;
He has made a decree which shall not pass away."
                  Psalm 119:89-91; 135:6; 148:5, 6.

It is not by inherent power that year by year the earth yields its bounties and continues its march around the sun. The hand of the Infinite One
is perpetually at work guiding this planet. It is God's power continually
exercised that keeps the earth in position in its rotation. It is God who
causes the sun to rise in the heavens. He opens the windows of heaven
and gives rain.

"He gives snow like wool;
He scatters the frost like ashes."

"When He utters His voice,
There is a multitude of waters in the heavens:
'And He causes the vapors to ascend from the ends of the
      earth.
He makes lightning for the rain,
He brings the wind out of His treasuries.'"
                  Psalm 147:16; Jeremiah 10:13.

It is by His power that vegetation flourishes, that every leaf appears,
every flower blooms, every fruit develops.

The mechanism of the human body cannot be fully understood. It
presents mysteries that baffle the most intelligent. The pulse beats, and
breath follows breath, but not as the result of a mechanism that, once
set in motion, continues its work. In God we live and move and have
our being. The beating heart, the throbbing pulse, every nerve and
muscle in the living organism, is kept in order and activity by the power
of an ever-present God.

The Bible shows us God in His high and holy place, not in a state of inactivity, not in silence and solitude, but surrounded by ten thousand times ten thousand and thousands of thousands of holy beings, all waiting to do His will. Through these messengers He is in active communication with every part of His dominion. By His Spirit He is everywhere present. Through the agency of His Spirit and His angels He ministers to His earthly children.

Above the distractions of the earth He sits enthroned. All things are open to His divine survey, and from His great and calm eternity He orders that which His providence sees best.

"The way of man is not in himself;
It is not in man who walks to direct his own steps."

"Trust in the Lord with all your heart. . . .
In all your ways acknowledge Him,
And He shall direct your paths."

"The eye of the Lord is on those who fear Him,
On those who hope in His mercy,
To deliver their soul from death,
And to keep them alive in famine."

"How precious is Your lovingkindness, O God! . . .
The children of men put their trust under the shadow
      of Your wings."
"Happy is he who has the God of Jacob for his help,
Whose hope is in the Lord his God."

"The earth, O Lord, is full of Your mercy."
You love "righteousness and justice."
You "are the confidence of all the ends of the earth,
And of the far-off seas;
Who established the mountains by His strength,
Being clothed with power;
You who still the noise of the seas, . . .
And the tumult of the peoples."

"You make the outgoings of the morning and evening
      rejoice."
"You crown the year with Your goodness,
And Your paths drip with abundance."

"The Lord upholds all who fall,
And raises up all who are bowed down.
The eyes of all look expectantly to You,
And You give them their food in due season.
You open Your hand
And satisfy the desire of every living thing."
> Jeremiah 10:23; Proverbs 3:5, 6; Psalm 33:18, 19;
> 36:7; 146:5; 119:64; 33:5; 65:5-7, 8, 11; 145:14-16.

Personality of God Revealed in Christ

In His Son, God has revealed Himself as a personal being. The outshining of the Father's glory "and the express image of His person," Jesus, as a personal Savior, came to the world. As a personal Savior He ascended on high. As a personal Savior He intercedes in the heavenly courts. Before the throne of God "One like the Son of Man" ministers in our behalf. Hebrews 1:3; Revelation 1:13.

Christ, the Light of the world, veiled the dazzling splendor of His divinity and came to live as a man among men, that mortals might, without being consumed, become acquainted with their Creator. Since sin brought separation between human beings and their Maker, no one has seen God at any time, except as He is manifested through Christ. "'I and My Father are one,'" Christ declared. "'No one knows the Son except the Father. Nor does anyone know the Father except the Son, and he to whom the Son wills to reveal Him.'" John 10:30; Matthew 11:27.

Christ came to teach us what God desires us to know. In the heavens above, in the earth, in the broad waters of the ocean, we see the handiwork of God. All created things testify to His power, His wisdom, His love.

Yet not from the stars or the ocean or the cataract can we learn of the personality of God as it was revealed in Christ. God saw that a clearer revelation than nature was needed to portray both His personality and His character. He sent His Son into the world to manifest, so far as human sight could endure, the nature and attributes of the invisible God.

Revealed to the Disciples

Let us study the words that Christ spoke in the upper chamber on the night before His crucifixion. He was nearing His hour of trial, and He sought to comfort His disciples, who were to be severely tempted and tried.

"'Let not your heart be troubled,'" He said. "'You believe in God, believe also in Me. In My Father's house are many mansions; if it were not so, I would have told you. I go to prepare a place for you.' . . .

"Thomas said to Him, 'Lord, we do not know where You are going, and how can we know the way?' Jesus said to him, 'I am the way, the truth, and the life. No one comes to the Father except through Me. If you had known Me, you would have known My Father also; and from now on you know Him and have seen Him.' . . .

" 'Lord, show us the Father,'" said Philip, " 'and it is sufficient for us.' Jesus said to him, 'Have I been with you so long, and yet you have not known Me, Philip? He who has seen Me has seen the Father; so how can you say, "Show us the Father"? Do you not believe that I am in the Father, and the Father in Me? The words that I speak to you I do not speak on My own authority; but the Father who dwells in Me does the works.'" John 14:1-10.

The disciples did not yet understand Christ's words concerning His relation to God. Much of His teaching was still obscure to them. Christ desired them to have a clearer, more distinct knowledge of God.

" 'These things I have spoken to you in figurative language,'" He said, " 'but the time is coming when I will no longer speak to you in figurative language, but I will tell you plainly about the Father.'" John 16:25.

On the Day of Pentecost, when the Holy Spirit was poured out on the disciples, they understood more fully the truths that Christ had spoken in figurative language. Much of the teaching that had been a mystery to them was made clear. But not even then did the disciples receive the complete fulfillment of Christ's promise. They received all the knowledge of God that they could bear, but the complete fulfillment of the promise that Christ would tell them plainly of the Father was yet to come.

Thus it is today. Our knowledge of God is partial and imperfect. When the conflict is ended, and the Man Christ Jesus acknowledges before the Father His faithful workers who in a world of sin have borne true witness for Him, they will understand clearly what now are mysteries to them.

Christ took with Him to the heavenly courts His glorified humanity. To those who receive Him He gives power to become sons and daughters of God, that at last God may receive them as His, to be with Him through-out eternity. If during this life they are loyal to God, they will at last "see His face, and His name shall be on their foreheads." Revelation 22:4. And what is the happiness of heaven but to see God? What greater joy could come to the sinner saved by the grace of Christ than to look upon the face of God and know Him as Father?

The Scriptures clearly indicate the relation between God and Christ, and they bring to view as clearly the personality and individuality of each.

"God, who at various times and in different ways spoke in time past to the fathers by the prophets, has in these last days spoken to us by His Son, . . . who being the brightness of His glory and the express image of His person, and upholding all things by the word of His power, when He had by Himself purged our sins, sat down at the right hand of the Majesty on high, having become so much better than the angels, as He has by inheritance obtained a more excellent name than they. For to which of the angels did He ever say:

> "'You are My Son,
> Today I have begotten You'?
> And again:
> 'I will be to Him a Father,
> And He shall be to Me a Son'?"
> Hebrews 1:1-5.

The personality of the Father and the Son, also the unity that exists between Them, are presented in the seventeenth chapter of John, in the prayer of Christ for His disciples: "'I do not pray for these alone, but also for those who will believe in Me through their word; that they all may be one, as You, Father, are in Me, and I in You; that they also may be one in Us, that the world may believe that You sent Me.'" John 17:20, 21.

The unity that exists between Christ and His disciples does not destroy the personality of either. They are one in purpose, in mind, in character, but not in person. It is thus that God and Christ are one.

Character of God Revealed in Christ

Taking humanity upon Him, Christ came to be one with humanity, and at the same time to reveal our heavenly Father to sinful human beings. Only He who had been in the presence of the Father from the beginning, only He who was the express image of the invisible God, was able to reveal the character of the Deity to humankind. In all things He was made like us. He became flesh even as we are. He was hungry and thirsty and weary. He was sustained by food and refreshed by sleep. He shared the lot of human beings, yet He was the blameless Son of God. He was a stranger and sojourner on the earth—in the world but not of the world, tempted and tried as men and women today are tempted and tried, yet living a life free from sin. Tender, compassionate, sympathetic, ever considerate of others, He represented the character of God and was constantly engaged in service for God and humanity.

> "'The Lord has anointed Me,'" He said,
> "'To preach good tidings to the poor;
> He has sent Me to heal the brokenhearted,
> To proclaim liberty to the captives,'"
> "'And recovery of sight to the blind;'"
> "'To proclaim the acceptable year of the Lord, . . .
> To comfort all who mourn.'"
> Isaiah 61:1; Luke 4:18; Isaiah 61:2.

"'Love your enemies,'" He bids us; "'bless those who curse you, do good to those who hate you, and pray for those who spitefully use you and persecute you, that you may be sons of your Father in heaven;'" "'for He is kind to the unthankful and evil.'" "'He makes His sun rise on the evil and on the good, and sends rain on the just and on the unjust.'" "'Therefore be merciful, just as your Father also is merciful.'" Matthew 5:44, 45; Luke 6:35; Matthew 5:45; Luke 6:36.

"'Through the tender mercy of our God, . . .
The Dayspring from on high has visited us;
To give light to those who sit in darkness and the
    shadow of death,
To guide our feet into the way of peace.'"
Luke 1:78, 79.

The Glory of the Cross

The revelation of God's love to us centers in the cross. Its full significance tongue cannot utter, pen cannot portray, the human mind cannot comprehend. Looking upon the cross of Calvary, we can only say, "God so loved the world that He gave His only begotten Son, that whoever believes in Him should not perish but have everlasting life." John 3:16.

Christ crucified for our sins, Christ risen from the dead, Christ ascended on high, is the science of salvation that we are to learn and to teach.

It was Christ "Who, existing in the form of God, counted not the being on an equality with God a thing to be grasped, but emptied Himself, taking the form of a servant, being made in the likeness of men; and being found in fashion as a man, He humbled Himself, becoming obedient even unto death, yea, the death of the cross." Philippians 2:6-8, ARV.

"It is Christ who died, and furthermore is also risen, who is even at the right hand of God." "Therefore He is also able to save to the uttermost those who come to God through Him, since He ever lives to make intercession for them." Romans 8:34; Hebrews 7:25.

"We do not have a High Priest who cannot sympathize with our weaknesses, but was in all points tempted as we are, yet without sin." Hebrews 4:15.

It is through the gift of Christ that we receive every blessing. Through that Gift there comes to us day by day the unfailing flow of God's goodness. Every flower, with its delicate tints and its fragrance, is given for our enjoyment through that one Gift. The sun and the moon were made by Him. There is not a star that beautifies the heavens that He did not make. Every drop of rain that falls, every ray of light shed upon our unthankful world, testifies to the love of God in Christ. Everything is supplied to us through the one unspeakable Gift, God's only-begotten Son. He was nailed to the cross that all these bounties might flow to God's workmanship.

"Behold what manner of love the Father has bestowed on us, that we should be called children of God!" 1 John 3:1.

"Men have not heard nor perceived by the ear,
Nor has the eye seen any God besides You,
Who acts for the one who waits for Him."
Isaiah 64:4.

The Knowledge That Works Transformation

The knowledge of God as revealed in Christ is the knowledge that all who are saved must have. It is the knowledge that works transformation of character. This knowledge, received, will re-create the soul in the image of God. It will impart to the whole being a spiritual power that is divine.

"We all, with unveiled face, beholding as in a mirror the glory of the Lord, are being transformed into the same image from glory to glory." 2 Corinthians 3:18.

Of His own life the Savior said, "'I have kept My Father's commandments.'" John 15:10. "'The Father has not left Me alone, for I always do those things that please Him.'" John 8:29. As Jesus was in human nature, so God means His followers to be. In His strength we are to live the life of purity and nobility that the Savior lived.

"For this reason," Paul says, "I bow my knees to the Father of our Lord Jesus Christ, from whom the whole family in heaven and earth is named, that He would grant you, according to the riches of His glory, to be strengthened with might through His Spirit in the inner man, that Christ may dwell in your hearts through faith; that you, being rooted and grounded in love, may be able to comprehend with all the saints what is the width and length and depth and height—to know the love of Christ which passes knowledge; that you may be filled with all the fullness of God." Ephesians 3:14-19.

We "do not cease to pray for you, and to ask that you may be filled with the knowledge of His will in all wisdom and spiritual understanding; that you may have a walk worthy of the Lord, fully pleasing Him, being fruitful in every good work and increasing in the knowledge of God; strengthened with all might, according to His glorious power, for all patience and longsuffering with joy." Colossians 1:9-11.

This is the knowledge that God is inviting us to receive, and beside which all else is vanity and nothingness.

Chapter 36

Danger in Speculative Knowledge

One of the greatest evils that attends the quest for knowledge, the investigations of science, is the disposition to exalt human reason above its true value and proper sphere. Many attempt to judge the Creator and His works by their own imperfect knowledge of science. They endeavor to determine the nature and attributes and prerogatives of God, indulging in speculative theories concerning the Infinite One. Those who engage in this line of study are treading on forbidden ground. Their research will yield no valuable results and can be pursued only at the peril of the soul.

Our first parents were led into sin through indulging a desire for knowledge that God had withheld from them. In seeking to gain this knowledge, they lost all that was worth possessing. If Adam and Eve had never touched the forbidden tree, God would have imparted to them knowledge—knowledge upon which rested no curse of sin, knowledge that would have brought them everlasting joy. All that they gained by listening to the tempter was an acquaintance with sin and its results. By their disobedience, humanity was estranged from God and the earth was separated from heaven.

The lesson is for us. The field into which Satan led our first parents is the same to which he is alluring people today. He is flooding the world with pleasing fables. By every device at his command he tempts men and women to speculate in regard to God. Thus he seeks to prevent them from obtaining that knowledge of God which is salvation.

Today there are coming into educational institutions and into the churches everywhere spiritualistic teachings that undermine faith in God and in His

Word. The theory that God is an essence pervading all nature is received by many who profess to believe the Scriptures, but however beautifully clothed, this theory is a most dangerous deception. It misrepresents God and is a dishonor to His greatness and majesty. It tends not only to mislead but to debase those who embrace it. Darkness is its element, sensuality its sphere. The result of accepting it is separation from God. And to fallen human nature this means ruin.

Our condition through sin is unnatural, and the power that restores us must be supernatural, or it has no value. There is only one power that can break the hold of evil from human hearts, and that is the power of God in Jesus Christ. Only through the blood of the Crucified One is there cleansing from sin. His grace alone can enable us to resist and subdue the tendencies of our fallen nature. Spiritualistic theories concerning God make His grace of no effect. If God is an essence pervading all nature, then He dwells in everybody, and in order to attain holiness, a person has only to develop the power within him or her.

These theories, followed to their logical conclusion, sweep away the whole Christian faith. They do away with the necessity for the atonement and make human beings their own savior. These theories regarding God make His Word of no effect, and those who accept them are in great danger of being led finally to look upon the whole Bible as fiction. They may regard virtue as better than vice, but, having shut out God from His rightful position of sovereignty, they place their dependence upon human power, which, without God, is worthless. The unaided human will has no real power to resist and overcome evil. The defenses of the soul are broken down. A person has no barrier against sin. When once the restraints of God's Word and His Spirit are rejected, who knows to what depths one may sink!

"Every word of God is pure;
He is a shield to those who put their trust in Him.
Do not add to His words,
Lest He rebuke you, and you be found a liar."

"His own iniquities entrap the wicked man,
And he is caught in the cords of his sin."
                              Proverbs 30:5, 6; 5:22.

Searching Into Divine Mysteries

"'The secret things belong to the Lord our God, but those things which are revealed belong to us and to our children forever.'" Deuteronomy 29:29. The revelation of Himself that God has given in His Word is for our study. This we may seek to understand. But beyond this we are not to penetrate. The highest intellect may tax itself until it is exhausted by conjecturing regarding the nature of God, but the effort will be fruitless. This problem has not been given us to solve. No human mind can comprehend God. None are to indulge in speculation regarding His nature. Here silence is eloquence. The Omniscient One is above discussion.

Even the angels were not permitted to share the counsels between the Father and the Son when the plan of salvation was laid. And human beings are not to intrude into the secrets of the Most High. We are as ignorant of God as little children, but, as little children, we may love and obey Him.

Instead of speculating in regard to His nature or His prerogatives, let us give heed to the words He has spoken:

> "'Can you search out the deep things of God?
> Can you find out the limits of the Almighty?
> They are higher than heaven—what can you do?
> Deeper than Sheol—what can you know?
> Their measure is longer than the earth
> And broader than the sea.'"

> "'Where can wisdom be found?
> And where is the place of understanding?
> Man does not know its value,
> Nor is it found in the land of the living.
> The deep says, "It is not in me";
> And the sea says, "It is not with me."
> It cannot be purchased for gold,
> Nor can silver be weighed for its price.
> It cannot be valued in the gold of Ophir,
> In precious onyx or sapphire. . . .

> " ' From where then does wisdom come?
> And where is the place of understanding? . . .
> Destruction and Death say,
> "We have heard a report about it with our ears."
> God understands its way,
> And He knows its place.
> For He looks to the ends of the earth,
> And sees under the whole heavens. . . .
> When He made a law for the rain,
> And a path for the thunderbolt,
> Then He saw wisdom and declared it;
> He prepared it, indeed, He searched it out.
> And to man He said,
> "Behold, the fear of the Lord, that is wisdom,
> And to depart from evil is understanding."'"
> Job 11:7-9; 28:12-28.

Deep Mysteries of God

Wisdom is not found by searching the recesses of the earth or in vain endeavors to penetrate the mysteries of God's being. It is found, rather, in humbly receiving the revelation that He has been pleased to give, and in conforming the life to His will.

Men and women of the greatest intellect cannot understand the mysteries of God as revealed in nature. Divine inspiration asks many questions that the most profound scholar cannot answer. These questions were not asked that we might answer them. They were asked to call our attention to the deep mysteries of God, to teach us that our wisdom is limited, and that in the surroundings of our daily life there are many things beyond the comprehension of finite beings.

Skeptics refuse to believe in God because they cannot comprehend the infinite power by which He reveals Himself. But God is to be acknowledged as much from what He does not reveal of Himself as from that which is open to our limited comprehension. Both in divine revelation and in nature, God has given mysteries to command our faith. This must be so. We may be ever searching, ever inquiring, ever learning, and yet there is an infinity beyond.

> "Who has measured the waters in the hollow of his hand,
> Measured heaven with a span
> And calculated the dust of the earth in a measure?
> Weighed the mountains in scales
> And the hills in a balance?
> Who has directed the Spirit of the Lord,
> Or as His counselor has taught Him? . . .
>
> "Behold, the nations are as a drop in a bucket,
> And are counted as the small dust on the balance;
> Look, He lifts up the isles as a very little thing.
> And Lebanon is not sufficient to burn,
> Nor its beasts sufficient for a burnt offering.
> All nations before Him are as nothing,
> And they are counted by Him less than nothing and worthless.
>
> "To whom then will you liken God?
> Or what likeness will you compare to Him? . . .
> Have you not known?
> Have you not heard?
> Has it not been told you from the beginning?
> Have you not understood from the foundations of the earth?
> It is He who sits above the circle of the earth,

And its inhabitants are like grasshoppers;
Who stretches out the heavens like a curtain,
And spreads them out like a tent to dwell in. . . .

" 'To whom then will you liken Me?' . . .
Says the Holy One.
Lift up your eyes on high,
And see who has created these things,
Who brings out their host by number;
He calls them all by name,
By the greatness of His might
And the strength of His power;
Not one is missing.

"Why do you say, O Jacob, and speak, O Israel:
'My way is hidden from the Lord,
And my just claim is passed over by my God'?
Have you not known?
Have you not heard?
The everlasting God, the Lord,
The Creator of the ends of the earth,
Neither faints nor is weary.
There is no searching of His understanding."
Isaiah 40:12-28.

Learning of God's Greatness

From the representations given by the Holy Spirit to His prophets, let us learn the greatness of our God. The prophet Isaiah writes:

"In the year that King Uzziah died, I saw the Lord sitting on a throne, high and lifted up, and the train of His robe filled the temple. Above it stood seraphim; each one had six wings: with two he covered his face, with two he covered his feet, and with two he flew. And one cried to another and said: 'Holy, holy, holy, is the Lord of hosts; the whole earth is full of His glory!' And the posts of the door were shaken by the voice of him who cried out, and the house was filled with smoke.

"Then I said, 'Woe is me, for I am undone! Because I am a man of unclean lips, and I dwell in the midst of a people of unclean lips; for my eyes have seen the King, the Lord of hosts.'

"Then one of the seraphim flew to me, having in his hand a live coal which he had taken with the tongs from the altar. And he touched my mouth with it, and said: 'Behold, this has touched your lips; your iniquity is taken away, and your sin purged.'" Isaiah 6:1-7.

"There is none like You, O Lord
(You are great, and Your name is great in might),
Who would not fear You, O King of the nations?"

"O Lord, You have searched me and known me.
You know my sitting down and my rising up;
You understand my thought afar off.
You comprehend my path and my lying down,
And are acquainted with all my ways.
For there is not a word on my tongue,
But behold, O Lord, You know it altogether.
You have hedged me behind and before,
And laid Your hand upon me.
Such knowledge is too wonderful for me;
It is high, I cannot attain it.' "
                    Jeremiah 10:6, 7; Psalm 139:1-6.

"Great is our Lord, and mighty in power; His understanding is infinite." Psalm 147:5.

"The ways of man are before the eyes of the Lord, and He ponders all his paths." Proverbs 5:21.

" 'He reveals deep and secret things; He knows what is in the darkness, and light dwells with Him.' " Daniel 2:22.

" 'Known to God from eternity are all His works.' " " 'Who has known the mind of the Lord? Or who has become His counselor?' 'Or who has first given to Him, and it shall be repaid to him?' For of Him and through Him and to Him are all things, to whom be glory forever." Acts 15:18; Romans 11:34-36.

"To the King eternal, immortal, invisible," "who alone has immortality, dwelling in unapproachable light, whom no man has seen or can see, to whom be honor and everlasting power." 1 Timothy 1:17; 6:16.

" 'Will not His excellence make you afraid,
And the dread of Him fall upon you?' "
" 'Is not God in the height of heaven?
And see the highest stars, how lofty they are!' "
" 'Is there any number to His armies?
Upon whom does His light not rise?' "
" 'He does great things which we cannot comprehend.
For He says to the snow, "Be on the earth";
Likewise to the gentle rain and the heavy rain of His strength.
He seals the hand of every man,
That all men may know His work. . . .
He scatters His bright clouds.

And they swirl about, being turned by His guidance,
That they may do whatever He commands them
On the face of the whole earth.
He causes it to come,
Whether for correction,
Or for His land,
Or for mercy. . . .

" 'Teach us what we should say to Him,
For we can prepare nothing because of the darkness. . . .
Even now men cannot look at the light when it is bright in the skies,
When the wind has passed and cleared them.
He comes from the north as golden splendor;
With God is awesome majesty.
As for the Almighty, we cannot find Him;
He is excellent in power,
In judgment and abundant justice; . . .
Therefore men fear Him.' "

"Who is like the Lord our God,
Who dwells on high,
Who humbles Himself to behold
The things that are in the heavens and in the earth?"

"The Lord has His way
In the whirlwind and in the storm,
And the clouds are the dust of His feet."

"Great is the Lord, and greatly to be praised;
And His greatness is unsearchable.
One generation shall praise Your works to another,
And shall declare Your mighty acts.
I will meditate on the glorious splendor of Your majesty,
And on Your wondrous works.
Men shall speak of the might of Your awesome acts,
And I will declare Your greatness.
They shall utter the memory of Your great goodness,
And shall sing of Your righteousness. . . .
"All Your works shall praise You, O Lord,
And Your saints shall bless You.
They shall speak of the glory of Your kingdom,
And talk of Your power,
To make known to the sons of men His mighty acts,

And the glorious majesty of His kingdom.
Your kingdom is an everlasting kingdom,
And Your dominion endures throughout all generations. . . .
My mouth shall speak the praise of the Lord,
And all flesh shall bless His holy name
Forever and ever."
>   Job 13:11; 22:12; 25:3; 37:5-13, 19-24;
>   Psalm 113:5, 6; Nahum 1:3; Psalm 145:3-21.

Lessons From Sacred History

As we learn more and more of what God is, and of what we ourselves are in His sight, we shall fear and tremble before Him. Let mortals of today take warning from the fate of those who in ancient times presumed to make free with that which God had declared sacred. When the Israelites ventured to open the ark on its return from the land of the Philistines, their irreverent daring was signally punished.

Again, consider the judgment that fell upon Uzzah. As in David's reign the ark was being carried to Jerusalem, Uzzah put forth his hand to keep it steady. For presuming to touch the symbol of God's presence, he was smitten with instant death.

At the burning bush, when Moses, not recognizing God's presence, turned aside to see the wonderful sight, the command was given: "'Do not draw near this place. Take your sandals off your feet, for the place where you stand is holy ground.' . . . And Moses hid his face, for he was afraid to look upon God." Exodus 3:5, 6.

"Now Jacob went out from Beersheba and went toward Haran. So he came to a certain place and stayed there all night, because the sun had set. And he took one of the stones of that place and put it at his head, and he lay down in that place to sleep.

"Then he dreamed, and behold, a ladder was set up on the earth, and its top reached to heaven, and there the angels of God were ascending and descending on it. And behold, the Lord stood above it and said: 'I am the Lord God of Abraham your father and the God of Isaac; the land on which you lie I will give to you and to your descendants. . . . Behold, I am with you and will keep you wherever you go, and will bring you back to this land; for I will not leave you until I have done what I have spoken to you.'

"Then Jacob awoke from his sleep and said, 'Surely the Lord is in this place, and I did not know it.' And he was afraid and said, 'How awesome is this place! This is none other than the house of God, and this is the gate of heaven!'" Genesis 28:10-17.

In the sanctuary of the wilderness tabernacle and of the temple that were the earthly symbols of God's dwelling place, one apartment was sacred to His presence. The veil inwrought with cherubim at its entrance was not to be lifted by any hand except one—that of the high priest. To lift that veil, and intrude unbidden into the sacred mystery of the most holy place, was death. For above the mercy seat appeared the glory of the Holiest—glory upon which no human might look and live. On the one day of the year appointed for ministry in the most holy place, the high priest with trembling entered God's presence, while clouds of incense veiled the glory from his sight. Throughout the courts of the temple every sound was hushed. No priests ministered at the altars. The host of worshipers, bowed in silent awe, offered their petitions for God's mercy.

"These things happened to them as examples, and they were written for our admonition, upon whom the ends of the ages have come." 1 Corinthians 10:11.

"'The Lord is in His holy temple.
Let all the earth keep silence before Him.' "

"The Lord reigns;
Let the peoples tremble!
He dwells between the cherubim;
Let the earth be moved!
The Lord is great in Zion,
And He is high above all the peoples.
Let them praise Your great and awesome name—
He is holy."

"He looked down from the height of His sanctuary."
"From the place of His habitation He looks
On all the inhabitants of the earth;
He fashions their hearts individually;
He considers all their works."
"Let all the earth fear the Lord;
Let all the inhabitants of the world stand in awe of Him."
   Habakkuk 2:20; Psalm 99:1-3; 102:19; 33:14, 15, 8.

Human beings cannot by searching find out God. Let none seek with presumptuous hand to lift the veil that conceals His glory. "Unsearchable are His judgments and His ways past finding out." Romans 11:33. It is a proof of His mercy that He hides His power, for to lift the veil that conceals the divine presence is death. No mortal mind can penetrate the secrecy in which the Mighty One dwells and works. Only that which He sees fit to reveal can we comprehend of Him. Reason must acknowledge an authority superior to itself. Heart and intellect must bow to the great I AM.

C h a p t e r   37

The False and the True in Education

The mastermind in the confederacy of evil is ever working to keep out of sight the words of God and to bring human opinions into view. He tries to keep us from hearing the voice of God saying, "'This is the way, walk in it.'" Isaiah 30:21. Through perverted educational processes he is doing his utmost to obscure heaven's light.

Philosophical speculation and scientific research in which God is not acknowledged are making skeptics of thousands. In the schools of today the conclusions that learned men and women have reached as the result of their scientific investigations are carefully taught and fully explained, and the impression is distinctly given that if these learned people are correct, the Bible cannot be. Skepticism is attractive to the human mind. The youth see in it an independence that captivates the imagination, and they are deceived. Satan triumphs. He nourishes every seed of doubt that is sown in young hearts. He causes it to grow and bear fruit, and soon a plentiful harvest of infidelity is reaped.

Because the human heart is inclined to evil, it is dangerous to sow seeds of skepticism in young minds. Whatever weakens faith in God robs the soul of power to resist temptation. It removes the only real safeguard against sin. We are in need of schools where the youth shall be taught that greatness consists in honoring God by revealing His character in daily life. Through His Word and His works we need to learn of God, that our lives may fulfill His purpose.

Infidel Authors

In order to obtain an education, many think it essential to study the writings of infidel authors, because these works contain many bright gems of thought. But who was the originator of these gems of thought? It was God, and God only. He is the source of all light. Why then should we wade through the mass of error contained in the works of infidels for the sake of a few intellectual truths, when all truth is at our command?

How is it that human beings who are at war with the government of God come into possession of the wisdom that they sometimes display? Satan himself was educated in the heavenly courts, and he has a knowledge of good as well as of evil. He mingles the precious with the vile, and this is what gives him power to deceive. But because Satan has robed himself in garments of heavenly brightness, shall we receive him as an angel of light? The tempter has his agents, educated according to his methods, inspired by his spirit, and adapted to his work. Shall we cooperate with them? Shall we receive the works of his agents as essential to the acquirement of an education?

If the time and effort spent in seeking to grasp the bright ideas of infidels were given to studying the precious things of the Word of God, thousands who now sit in darkness and in the shadow of death would be rejoicing in the glory of the Light of life.

Historical and Theological Lore

As a preparation for Christian work, many think it essential to acquire an extensive knowledge of historical and theological writings. They suppose that this knowledge will be an aid to them in teaching the gospel. But their laborious study of human opinions tends to enfeeble their ministry rather than strengthen it.

As I see libraries filled with ponderous volumes of historical and theological lore, I think, "'Why do you spend money for what is not bread?'" Isaiah 55:2. The sixth chapter of John tells us more than can be found in such works. Christ says: "'I am the Bread of Life. He who comes to Me shall never hunger, and he who believes in Me shall never thirst.'" "'I am the living Bread which came down from heaven. If anyone eats of this Bread, he will live forever.'" "'He who believes in Me has everlasting life.'" "'The words that I speak to you are spirit, and they are life.'" John 6:35, 51, 47, 63.

There is a study of history that is not to be condemned. Sacred history was one of the studies in the schools of the prophets. In the record of God's dealings with the nations were traced His footsteps. So today we are to consider the dealings of God with the nations of the earth. We are to see in history the fulfillment of prophecy. We are to study the workings of Providence in the great reformatory movements and to understand the progress of events in the marshaling of the nations for the final conflict of the great controversy.

Such study will give broad, comprehensive views of life. It will help us to understand something of its relations and dependencies, how wonderfully we are bound together in the great community of society and nations, and to how great an extent the oppression and degradation of one member means loss to all.

But history, as commonly studied, is concerned with human achievements such as victories in battle and success in attaining power and greatness. God's agency in human affairs is lost sight of. Few study the working out of His purpose in the rise and fall of nations.

And, to a great degree, theology, as studied and taught, is but a record of human speculation, serving only to "darken counsel by words without knowledge." Job 38:2. Too often the motive in accumulating these many books is not a desire to obtain food for mind and soul, it is an ambition to become acquainted with philosophers and theologians, a desire to present Christianity to the people in learned terms and propositions.

Not all the books written can serve the purpose of a holy life. "'Learn from Me,'" said the Great Teacher, "'take My yoke upon you,' learn My meekness and lowliness." Your intellectual pride will not aid you in communicating with souls who are perishing for want of the bread of life. In your study of these books you are allowing them to take the place of the practical lessons you should be learning from Christ. The results of this study do not feed the people. Very little of the research that is so wearying to the mind furnishes help for a person who wants to be a successful soul winner.

The Savior came "'to preach the gospel to the poor.'" Luke 4:18. In His teaching He used the simplest terms and the plainest symbols. And it is said that "the common people heard Him gladly." Mark 12:37. Those who are seeking to do His work for this time need a deeper insight into the lessons He has given.

The words of the living God are the highest of all education. Those who minister to the people need to eat of the Bread of Life. This will give them spiritual strength. Then they will be prepared to minister to all classes of people.

The Classics

In the colleges and universities thousands of youth devote a large part of the best years of life to the study of Greek and Latin. And while they are engaged in these studies, mind and character are molded by the evil sentiments of pagan literature, the reading of which is generally regarded as an essential part of the study of these languages.

Those who are familiar with the classics declare that "the Greek tragedies are full of incest, murder, and human sacrifices to lustful and revengeful gods." It would be far better for the world if the education gained from such sources were to be dispensed with. "Can one walk on hot coals, and his feet not be seared?" Proverbs 6:28. "'Who can bring a clean thing out of an unclean? No one!'" Job 14:4. Can we then expect the youth to develop Christian character while their education is molded by the teaching of those who set at defiance the principles of the law of God?

In casting off restraint and plunging into reckless amusement, dissipation, and vice, students are but imitating that which is kept before their minds by these studies. There are callings in which a knowledge of Greek and Latin is needed. Some must study these languages. But the knowledge of them essential for practical uses might be gained without a study of literature that is corrupt and corrupting.

And a knowledge of Greek and Latin is not needed by many. The study of dead languages should be made secondary to a study of those subjects that teach the right use of all the powers of body and mind. It is folly for students to devote their time to the acquirement of dead languages or of book knowledge in any line, to the neglect of a training for life's practical duties.

What do students carry with them when they leave school? Where are they going? What are they to do? Have they the knowledge that will enable them to teach others? Have they been educated to be good fathers and mothers? Can they stand at the head of a family as wise instructors? The only education worthy of the name is that which leads young men and young women to be Christlike, that fits them to bear life's responsibilities, fits them to stand at the head of their families. Such an education is not acquired by a study of heathen classics.

Sensational Literature

Many of the popular publications of the day are filled with sensational stories that are educating the youth in wickedness and leading them in the path to perdition. Mere children in years are old in a knowledge of crime. They are incited to evil by the tales they read. In imagination they act out the deeds portrayed, until their ambition is aroused to see what they can do in committing crime and evading punishment. To the active minds of children and youth the scenes pictured in imaginary revelations of the future are realities. As revolutions are predicted and all manner of proceedings described that break down the barriers of law and self-restraint, many catch the spirit of these representations. They are led to commit crimes even worse, if possible, than these sensational writers depict. Through influences such as these, society is becoming demoralized. The seeds of lawlessness are sown everywhere, and a harvest of crime is the result.

Works of romance, frivolous, exciting tales, are, in hardly less degree, a curse to the reader. Authors may profess to teach a moral lesson, they may interweave religious sentiments throughout their work, but often these serve only to veil the folly and worthlessness beneath.

The world is flooded with books that are filled with enticing error. The youth receive as truth that which the Bible denounces as falsehood, and they love and cling to deception that means ruin to the soul.

There are works of fiction that were written for the purpose of teaching truth or exposing some great evil. Some of these works have accomplished good. Yet they have also wrought untold harm. They contain statements and highly wrought pen pictures that excite the imagination and give rise to a train of thought that is full of danger, especially to the youth. The scenes described are lived over and over again in their thoughts. Such reading unfits the mind for usefulness and disqualifies it for spiritual exercise. It destroys interest in the Bible. Heavenly things find little place in the thoughts. As the mind dwells upon the scenes of impurity portrayed, passion is aroused, and the end is sin.

Even fiction that contains no suggestion of impurity, and which may be intended to teach excellent principles, is harmful. It encourages the habit of hasty and superficial reading merely for the story. Thus it tends to destroy the power of connected and vigorous thought. It unfits the soul to contemplate the great problems of duty and destiny.

By fostering love for mere amusement, the reading of fiction creates a distaste for life's practical duties. Through its exciting, intoxicating power it is not infrequently a cause of both mental and physical disease. Many a miserable, neglected home, many a lifelong invalid, many an inmate of the insane asylum, has become such through the habit of novel reading.

It is often urged that in order to win the youth from sensational or worthless literature we should supply them with a better class of fiction. This is like trying to cure an alcoholic by giving him the milder intoxicants, such as wine, beer, or cider, in the place of whisky or brandy. The use of these would continually foster the appetite for stronger stimulants. The only safety for an alcoholic, and the only safeguard for the temperate person, is total abstinence. For the lover of fiction the same rule holds true. Total abstinence is one's only safety.

Myths and Fairy Tales

In the education of children and youth, fairy tales, myths, and fictitious stories are now given a large place. Books of this character are used in schools, and they are to be found in many homes. How can Christian parents permit their children to use books filled with falsehood! When the children ask the meaning of stories so contrary to the teaching of their parents, the answer is that the stories are not true, but this does not do away with the evil results of their use. The ideas presented in these books mislead the children. They impart false views of life and create and foster a desire for the unreal.

The widespread use of such books at this time is one of the cunning devices of Satan. He is seeking to divert the minds of old and young from the great work of character building. He purposes that our children and youth shall be swept away by the soul-destroying deceptions with which he is filling the world. Therefore he seeks to divert their minds from the Word of God and thus prevent them from obtaining a knowledge of those truths that would be their safeguard.

Never should books containing a perversion of truth be placed in the hands of children or youth. Let not our children, in the very process of obtaining an education, receive ideas that will prove to be seeds of sin. Even people with mature minds would be far safer if they had nothing to do with such books, and their example and influence on the right side would make it much easier to guard the youth from temptation.

We have an abundance of that which is real, that which is divine. Those who thirst for knowledge need not go to polluted fountains. The Lord says:

"Incline your ear and hear the words of the wise,
And apply your heart to My knowledge. . . .
That your trust may be in the Lord;
I have instructed you today, even you.
Have I not written to you excellent things
Of counsels and knowledge,
That I may make you know the certainty of the words of truth,
That you may answer words of truth
To those who send to you?"

"He established a testimony in Jacob,
And appointed a law in Israel,
Which He commanded our fathers,
That they should make them known to their children;"
"Telling to the generation to come the praises of the Lord,
And His strength and His wonderful works that He has done."
"That the generation to come might know them,
The children who would be born,
That they may arise and declare them to their children,
That they may set their hope in God."
"The blessing of the Lord makes one rich,
And He adds no sorrow with it."
Proverbs 22:17-21; Psalm 78:5, 4, 6, 7; Proverbs 10:22.

Christ's Teaching

So also Christ presented the principles of truth in the gospel. In His teaching we may drink of the pure streams that flow from the throne of God. Christ could have imparted knowledge that would have surpassed any previous disclosures and put in the background every other discovery. He could have unlocked mystery after mystery, and could have concentrated around these wonderful revelations the active, earnest thought of successive generations till the close of time. But He would not spare a moment from teaching the science of salvation. His time, His faculties, and His life were appreciated and used only as a means of working for the salvation of souls. He had come to seek and to save that which was lost, and He would not be turned from His purpose. He allowed nothing to divert Him.

Christ imparted only knowledge that could be used. His instruction of the people was confined to the needs of their own condition in practical life. He did not gratify the curiosity that led them to come to Him with prying questions. He made all such questionings an occasion for solemn, earnest, vital appeals. To those who were so eager to pick fruit from the tree of knowledge, He offered the fruit of the tree of life. They found every avenue closed except the way that leads to God. Every fountain was sealed except the fountain of eternal life.

Our Savior did not encourage any to attend the rabbinical schools of His day, for the reason that their minds would be corrupted with the continually repeated, "They say . . ." or, "It has been said . . . ." Why, then, should we accept the unstable words of men and women as exalted wisdom, when a greater, a certain, wisdom is at our command?

That which I have seen of eternal things, and that which I have seen of the weakness of humanity, has deeply impressed my mind and influenced my lifework. I see nothing wherein mortals should be praised or glorified. I see no reason why the opinions of worldly-wise people and so-called great thinkers should be trusted and exalted. How can those who are destitute of divine enlightenment have correct ideas of God's plans and ways? They either deny Him altogether and ignore His existence, or they circumscribe His power by their own finite conceptions.

Let us choose to be taught by Him who created the heavens and the earth, by Him who set the stars in their order in the firmament and appointed the sun and the moon to do their work.

It is right for the youth to feel that they must reach the highest development of their mental powers. We would not restrict the education to which God has set no limit. But our attainments avail nothing if not put to use for the honor of God and the good of humanity.

It is not well to crowd the mind with studies that require intense application but that are not brought into use in practical life. Such education will be a loss to students. These studies lessen their desire and inclination for studies that would fit them for usefulness and enable them to fulfill their responsibilities. A practical training is worth far more than any amount of mere theorizing. It is not enough even to have knowledge. We must have ability to use the knowledge aright.

The time, means, and study that so many expend for a comparatively useless education should be devoted to gaining an education that would make them practical men and women, fitted to bear life's responsibilities. Such an education would be of the highest value.

What we need is knowledge that will strengthen mind and soul, that will make us better men and women. Heart education is of far more importance than mere book learning. It is well, even essential, to have a knowledge of the world in which we live, but if we leave eternity out of our reckoning we shall make a failure from which we can never recover.

Students may devote all their powers to acquiring knowledge, but unless they have a knowledge of God, unless they obey the laws that govern their own being, they will destroy themselves. By wrong habits, they lose the power of self-appreciation. They lose self-control. They cannot reason correctly about matters that concern them most deeply. They are reckless and irrational in their treatment of mind and body. Through their neglect to cultivate right principles, they are ruined both for this world and for the world to come.

If the youth understood their own weakness, they would find in God their strength. If they seek to be taught by Him, they will become wise in His wisdom and their lives will be fruitful of blessing to the world. But if they give up their minds to mere worldly and speculative study, and thus separate from God, they will lose all that enriches life.

The Importance of Seeking True Knowledge

We need to understand more clearly than we do the issues at stake in the great conflict in which we are engaged. We need to understand more fully the value of the truths of the Word of God and the danger of allowing our minds to be diverted from them by the great deceiver.

The infinite value of the sacrifice required for our redemption reveals the fact that sin is a tremendous evil. Through sin the whole human organism is deranged. The mind is perverted, the imagination corrupted. Sin has degraded the faculties of the soul. Temptations from without find an answering chord within the heart, and the feet turn imperceptibly toward evil.

As the sacrifice in our behalf was complete, so our restoration from the defilement of sin is to be complete. The law of God will not excuse any act of wickedness; no unrighteousness can escape its condemnation. The ethics of the gospel acknowledge no standard but the perfection of the divine character. The life of Christ was a perfect fulfillment of every precept of the law. He said, "'I have kept My Father's commandments.'" His life is our example of obedience and service. God alone can renew the heart. "It is God who works in you both to will and to do for His good pleasure." But we are bidden, "Work out your own salvation." John 15:10; Philippians 2:13, 12.

The Work That Requires Our Thought

Wrongs cannot be righted nor can reformations in conduct be made by a few feeble, intermittent efforts. Character building is the work, not of a day, nor of a year, but of a lifetime. The struggle for conquest over self, for holiness and heaven, is a lifelong struggle. Without continual effort and constant activity, there can be no advancement in the divine life, no attainment of the victor's crown.

The strongest evidence that humanity has fallen from a higher state is the fact that it costs so much to return. The way of return can be gained only by hard fighting, inch by inch, hour by hour. In one moment, by a hasty, unguarded act, we may place ourselves in the power of evil, but it requires more than a moment to break the fetters and attain to a holier life. The purpose may be formed, the process begun, but its accomplishment will require hard work, time, perseverance, patience, and sacrifice.

We cannot allow ourselves to act from impulse. We cannot be off guard for a moment. Faced with temptations without number, we must resist firmly or be conquered. If we were to come to the close of life with our work undone, it would be an eternal loss.

The life of the apostle Paul was a constant conflict with self. He said, "I die daily." 1 Corinthians 15:31. His will and his desires every day conflicted with duty and the will of God. But instead of following inclination, he did God's will, however crucifying to his nature.

At the close of his life of conflict, looking back over its struggles and triumphs, he could say, "I have fought the good fight, I have finished the race, I have kept the faith. Finally, there is laid up for me the crown of righteousness, which the Lord, the righteous Judge, will give me on that Day." 2 Timothy 4:7, 8.

The Christian life is a battle and a march. From this warfare there is no release. The effort must be continuous and persevering. It is by unceasing endeavor that we maintain the victory over the temptations of Satan. Christian integrity must be sought with resistless energy and maintained with a resolute fixedness of purpose.

No one will be borne upward without stern, persevering effort in his or her own behalf. All must engage in this warfare for themselves. No one else can fight our battles. Individually we are responsible for the issues of the struggle. Though Noah, Job, and Daniel were in the land, they could deliver neither son nor daughter by their righteousness. (See Ezekiel 14:12-20.)

The Science to Be Mastered

There is a science of Christianity to be mastered—a science as much deeper, broader, higher than any human science as the heavens are higher than the earth. The mind is to be disciplined, educated, and trained, for we are to do service for God in ways that are not in harmony with inborn inclination. Hereditary and cultivated tendencies to evil must be overcome.

Often the education and training of a lifetime must be discarded, that we may become learners in the school of Christ.

Our hearts must be educated to become steadfast in God. We are to form habits of thought that will enable us to resist temptation. We must learn to look upward. The principles of the Word of God—principles that are as high as heaven, and that compass eternity—we are to understand in their bearing upon our daily life. Every act, every word, every thought, is to be in accord with these principles. All must be brought into harmony with, and subject to, Christ.

The precious graces of the Holy Spirit are not developed in a moment. Courage, fortitude, meekness, faith, unwavering trust in God's power to save, are acquired by the experience of years. By a life of holy endeavor and firm adherence to the right, the children of God are to seal their destiny.

No Time to Lose

We have no time to lose. We do not know how soon our probation may close. At the longest, we have but a brief lifetime here, and we do not know how soon the arrow of death may strike our hearts. We do not know how soon we may be called to give up the world and all its interests. Eternity stretches before us. The curtain is about to be lifted. Soon the mandate will go forth for everyone now numbered with the living: "'He who is unjust, let him be unjust still; . . . he who is righteous, let him be righteous still; he who is holy, let him be holy still.'" Revelation 22:11.

Are we prepared? Have we become acquainted with God, the Governor of heaven, the Lawgiver, and with Jesus Christ whom He sent into the world as His representative? When our lifework is ended, shall we be able to say, as did Christ our example: "'I have glorified You on the earth. I have finished the work which You have given Me to do. . . . I have manifested Your name'"? John 17:4-6.

The angels of God are seeking to attract us from ourselves and from earthly things. May this work not be in vain.

Minds that have been given up to loose thought need to change. "Gird up the loins of your mind, be sober, and rest your hope fully upon the grace that is to be brought to you at the revelation of Jesus Christ; as obedient children, not conforming yourselves to the former lusts, as in your ignorance; but as He who called you is holy, you also be holy in all your conduct, because it is written, 'Be holy, for I am holy.'" 1 Peter 1:13-16.

The thoughts must be centered upon God. We must put forth earnest effort to overcome the evil tendencies of the natural heart. Our efforts, our self-denial and perseverance, must be proportionate to the infinite value of the object we are pursuing. Only by overcoming as Christ overcame shall we win the crown of life.

The Need of Self-renunciation

Our great danger is in being self-deceived, indulging self-sufficiency, and thus separating from God, the source of our strength. Our natural tendencies, unless corrected by the Holy Spirit of God, have in them the seeds of moral death. Unless we become vitally connected with God, we cannot resist the unhallowed effects of self-indulgence, self-love, and temptation to sin.

In order to receive help from Christ, we must realize our need. We must have a true knowledge of ourselves. Christ can save only those who know themselves to be sinners. Only as we see our utter helplessness and renounce all self-trust shall we lay hold on divine power.

It is not only at the beginning of the Christian life that this renunciation of self is to be made. At every advance step heavenward it is to be renewed. All our good works are dependent on a power outside of ourselves. Therefore there needs to be a continual reaching out of the heart after God, a constant, earnest confession of sin and humbling of the soul before Him. Perils surround us, and we are safe only as we feel our weakness and cling with the grasp of faith to our mighty Deliverer.

Christ the Fountainhead of True Knowledge

We must turn away from a thousand topics that invite attention. There are matters that consume time and arouse inquiry, but end in nothing. The highest interests of the soul demand the close attention and energy that are often given to comparatively insignificant things. Accepting new theories does not in itself bring new life to the soul. Even an acquaintance with facts and theories important in themselves is of little value unless put to practical use. We need to feel our responsibility to give our souls food that will nourish and stimulate spiritual life.

"Incline your ear to wisdom, . . .
Apply your heart to understanding; . . .
Seek her as silver, . . .
Search for her as for hidden treasures;
Then you will understand the fear of the Lord,
And find the knowledge of God. . . .
Then you will understand righteousness and justice,
Equity and every good path.
When wisdom enters your heart,
And knowledge is pleasant to your soul,
Discretion will preserve you;
Understanding will keep you."
Wisdom "is a tree of life to those who take hold of her,
And happy are all who retain her."
Proverbs 2:2-11; 3:18.

The question for us to study is, "What is truth—the truth that is to be cherished, loved, honored, and obeyed?" The devotees of science have been defeated and disheartened in their efforts to find out God. What they need to inquire at this time is, "What is the truth that will enable us to win the salvation of our souls?"

"What do you think of Christ?"—this is the all-important question. Do you receive Him as a personal Savior? To all who receive Him He gives power to become children of God.

Christ revealed God to His disciples in a way that performed in their hearts a special work, such as He desires to do in our hearts. There are many who, in dwelling too largely upon theory, have lost sight of the living power of the Savior's example. They have lost sight of Him as the humble, self-denying worker. What they need is to behold Jesus. Daily we need the fresh revealing of His presence. We need to follow more closely His example of self-renunciation and self-sacrifice.

We need the experience that Paul had when he wrote: "I have been crucified with Christ; it is no longer I who live, but Christ lives in me; and the life which I now live in the flesh I live by faith in the Son of God, who loved me and gave Himself for me." Galatians 2:20.

The knowledge of God and of Jesus Christ expressed in character is an exaltation above everything else that is esteemed on earth or in heaven. It is the very highest education. It is the key that opens the portals of the heavenly city. This knowledge it is God's purpose that all who put on Christ shall possess.

Chapter 39

The Knowledge Received Through God's Word

The whole Bible is a revelation of the glory of God in Christ. Received, believed, obeyed, it is the great instrumentality in the transformation of character. It is the grand stimulus, the constraining force, that quickens the physical, mental, and spiritual powers, and directs the life into right channels.

The reason why so many are easily led into temptation and sin is that they do not study the Word of God and meditate upon it as they should. They do not by earnest effort direct the mind to that which would inspire pure, holy thought and divert it from that which is impure and untrue. The lack of firm, decided will power, which is manifest in life and character, results from neglect of the sacred instruction of God's Word. There are few who choose the better part, who sit at the feet of Jesus, as did Mary, to learn of the divine Teacher. Few treasure His words in the heart and practice them in the life.

The truths of the Bible, received, will uplift mind and soul. If the Word of God were appreciated as it should be, both young and old would possess a moral backbone, a strength of principle that would enable them to resist temptation.

Let men and women teach and write the precious things of the Holy Scriptures. Let the thought, the aptitude, the keen exercise of brain power, be given to the study of the thoughts of God. Do not study the philosophy of human conjectures, but study the philosophy of Him who is truth. No other literature can compare with this in value.

The mind that is earthly finds no pleasure in contemplating the Word of God, but for the mind renewed by the Holy Spirit, divine beauty and celestial light shine from the sacred page. That which to the earthly mind is a desolate wilderness, to the spiritual mind becomes a land of living streams.

The knowledge of God as revealed in His Word is the knowledge to be given to our children. From the earliest dawn of reason, they should be made familiar with the name and the life of Jesus. Their first lessons should teach them that God is their Father. Their first training should be that of loving obedience. Reverently and tenderly let the Word of God be read and repeated to them in portions suited to their comprehension and adapted to awaken their interest. Above all, let them learn of God's love revealed in Christ, and its great lesson: "If God so loved us, we also ought to love one another." 1 John 4:11.

Young people should make the Word of God the food of mind and soul. The cross of Christ should be made the science of all education, the center of all teaching and all study. Let it be brought into the daily experience in practical life. In this way the Savior will become to the youth a daily companion and friend. Every thought will be brought into captivity to the obedience of Christ. With the apostle Paul they will be able to say: "God forbid that I should glory except in the cross of our Lord Jesus Christ, by whom the world has been crucified to me, and I to the world." Galatians 6:14.

Thus through faith they come to know God by an experimental knowledge. They have proved for themselves the reality of His Word, the truth of His promises. They have tasted, and they know that the Lord is good.

The beloved John had a knowledge gained through his own experience. He could testify: "That which was from the beginning, which we have heard, which we have seen with our eyes, which we have looked upon, and our hands have handled, concerning the Word of life—the life was manifested, and we have seen, and bear witness, and declare to you that eternal life which was with the Father and was manifested to us—that which we have seen and heard we declare to you, that you also may have fellowship with us; and truly our fellowship is with the Father and with His Son Jesus Christ." 1 John 1:1-3.

So all may be able, through their own experience, to certify that "God is true." John 3:33. They can bear witness to that which they themselves have seen and heard and felt of the power of Christ. They can testify: "I needed help, and I found it in Jesus. Every want was supplied. The hunger of my soul was satisfied. The Bible is to me the revelation of Christ. I believe in Jesus because He is to me a divine Savior. I believe the Bible because I have found it to be the voice of God to my soul."

Any man or woman who has gained a knowledge of God and His Word through personal experience is prepared to engage in the study of natural science. Of Christ it is written, "In Him was life, and the life was the light of men." John 1:4. Before the entrance of sin, Adam and Eve in Eden were surrounded with a clear and beautiful light, the light of God. This light illuminated everything that they approached. There was nothing to obscure their perception of the character or the works of God. But when they yielded to the tempter, the light departed from them. In losing the garments of holiness, they lost the light that had illuminated nature. No longer could they read it aright. They could not discern the character of God in His works.

So today human beings cannot of themselves read aright the teaching of nature. Unless guided by divine wisdom, they exalt nature and the laws of nature above nature's God. This is why mere human ideas in regard to science so often contradict the teaching of God's Word. But for those who receive the light of the life of Christ, nature is again illuminated. In the light shining from the cross, we can rightly interpret nature's teaching.

Those who have a knowledge of God and His Word through personal experience have a settled faith in the divinity of the Holy Scriptures. They have proved that God's Word is truth, and they know that truth can never contradict itself. They do not test the Bible by human ideas of science; they bring these ideas to the test of the unerring standard. They know that in true science there can be nothing contrary to the teaching of the Word. Since both have the same Author, a correct understanding of both will prove them to be in harmony. Whatever in so-called scientific teaching contradicts the testimony of God's Word is mere human guesswork.

To students with this outlook, scientific research will open vast fields of thought and information. As they contemplate the things of nature, they receive a new perception of truth. The book of nature and the written Word shed light upon each other. Both make them better acquainted with God by teaching them of His character and of the laws through which He works.

The experience of the psalmist is the experience that all may gain by receiving God's Word through nature and through revelation. He says:

"You, Lord, have made me glad through Your work;
I will triumph in the works of Your hands."
"Your mercy, O Lord, is in the heavens;
Your faithfulness reaches to the clouds.
Your righteousness is like the great mountains;
Your judgments are a great deep. . . .
How precious is Your lovingkindness, O God! . . .
The children of men put their trust under the
    shadow of Your wings. . . .
And You give them drink from the river of Your pleasures.
For with You is the fountain of life;
In Your light we see light."

"Blessed are the undefiled in the way,
Who walk in the law of the Lord!
Blessed are those who keep His testimonies,
Who seek Him with the whole heart!"

"How can a young man cleanse his way?
By taking heed according to Your word."
"I have chosen the way of truth;
Your judgments I have laid before me."
"Your word I have hidden in my heart,
That I might not sin against You."
"And I will walk at liberty;
For I seek Your precepts."

"Open my eyes, that I may see
Wondrous things from Your law."
"Your testimonies also are my delight
And my counselors."
"The law of Your mouth is better to me
Than thousands of shekels of gold and silver."

"Oh, how I love Your law!
It is my meditation all the day."
"Your testimonies are wonderful;
Therefore my soul keeps them."
"Your statutes have been my songs
In the house of my pilgrimage."

"Your word is very pure;
Therefore Your servant loves it."

"The entirety of Your word is truth,
And every one of Your righteous judgments
    endures forever."

"Let my soul live, and it shall praise You;
And let Your judgments help me."
"Great peace have those who love Your law;
And nothing causes them to stumble.
Lord, I hope for Your salvation,
And I do Your commandments.
My soul keeps Your testimonies,
And I love them exceedingly."

"The entrance of Your words gives light;
It gives understanding to the simple."
"You, through Your commandments, make me wiser
     than my enemies;
For they are ever with me.
I have more understanding than all my teachers,
For Your testimonies are my meditation.
I understand more than the ancients,
Because I keep Your precepts."
"Through Your precepts I get understanding;
Therefore I hate every false way."

"Your testimonies I have taken as a heritage forever,
For they are the rejoicing of my heart."
          Psalm 92:4; 36:5-9; 119:1, 2, 9, 30, 11, 45, 18, 24,
72, 97, 129, 54, 140, 160, 175, 165-167, 130, 98-100, 104, 111.

Clearer Revelations of God

It is our privilege to reach higher and still higher for clearer revelations of the character of God. When Moses prayed, "'Please, show me Your glory,'" the Lord did not rebuke him; He granted his prayer. God declared to His servant, "'I will make all My goodness pass before you, and I will proclaim the name of the Lord before you.'" Exodus 33:18, 19.

Sin darkens the mind and dims our perceptions. As sin is purged from our hearts, the light of the knowledge of the glory of God in the face of Jesus Christ, illuminating His Word and reflected from the face of nature, more and more fully will declare Him "'merciful and gracious, longsuffering, and abounding in goodness and truth.'" Exodus 34:6.

In His light we shall see light, until mind and heart and soul are transformed into the image of His holiness.

For those who thus lay hold of the divine assurances of God's Word, there are wonderful possibilities. Before them lie vast fields of truth, vast resources of power. Glorious things are to be revealed. Privileges and duties that they do not even suspect to be in the Bible will be made manifest. All who walk in the path of humble obedience, fulfilling His purpose, will obtain more and more of the wisdom of God.

If students take the Bible as their guide and stand firmly for principle, they may aspire to any height of attainment. All the philosophies of human nature have led to confusion and shame when God has not been recognized as all in all. But the precious faith inspired of God imparts strength and nobility of character. As His goodness, His mercy, and His love are dwelt upon, clearer and still clearer will be the perception of truth. Higher, holier, will be the desire for purity of heart and clearness of thought. The soul dwelling in the pure atmosphere of holy thought is transformed by interacting with God through the study of His Word. Truth is so large, so far-reaching, so deep, so broad, that self is lost sight of. The heart is softened and subdued into humility, kindness, and love.

And the natural powers are enlarged because of holy obedience. From the study of the Word of life, students may come forth with minds expanded, elevated, ennobled. If, like Daniel, they are hearers and doers of the Word of God, they may advance as he did in all branches of learning. Being pure-minded, they will become strong-minded. Every intellectual faculty will be quickened. They may so educate and discipline themselves that all within the sphere of their influence shall see what a person can be and do when connected with the God of wisdom and power.

Education in the Future Life

Our lifework here is a preparation for the life eternal. The education begun here will not be completed in this life; it will go forward through all eternity—ever progressing, never completed. The wisdom and love of God in the plan of redemption will more and more fully be revealed. The Savior, as He leads His children to the fountains of living waters, will impart rich stores of knowledge. And day by day the wonderful works of God, the evidences of His power in creating and sustaining the universe, will open before the mind in new beauty. In the light that shines from the throne, mysteries will disappear and the soul will be filled with astonishment at the simplicity of the things that were never before comprehended.

"Now we see in a mirror, dimly, but then face to face. Now I know in part, but then I shall know just as I also am known." 1 Corinthians 13:12.

The Worker's Need

Chapter 40

Help in
Daily Living

There is an eloquence far more powerful than the eloquence of words in the quiet, consistent life of a pure, true Christian. What a person is has more influence than what he or she says.

The officers who were sent to Jesus came back with the report that no man had ever spoken as He spoke. But the reason for this was that no man had ever lived as He lived. If His life had been other than it was, He could not have spoken as He did. His words had convincing power because they came from a heart pure and holy, full of love and sympathy, benevolence and truth.

Our own character and experience determine our influence upon others. In order to convince others of the power of Christ's grace, we must know its power in our own hearts and lives. The gospel we present for the saving of souls must be the gospel by which our own souls are saved. Only through a living faith in Christ as a personal Savior is it possible to make our influence felt in a skeptical world. If we would draw sinners out of the swift-running current, our own feet must be firmly set upon the Rock, Christ Jesus.

The badge of Christianity is not an outward sign, not the wearing of a cross or a crown; it is that which reveals the union of the soul with God. By the power of His grace manifested in the transformation of character, the world is to be convinced that God has sent His Son as its Redeemer. No other influence that can surround a person has such power as the influence of an unselfish life. The strongest argument in favor of the gospel is a loving and lovable Christian.

The Discipline of Trial

To live such a life, to exert such an influence, costs at every step effort, self-sacrifice, discipline. Because they do not understand this, many are easily discouraged in the Christian life. Many who sincerely consecrate their lives to God's service are surprised and disappointed to find themselves, as never before, confronted by obstacles and beset by trials and perplexities. They pray for Christlikeness of character, for a fitness for the Lord's work, and then are placed in circumstances that seem to call forth all the evil of their nature. Faults are revealed of which they did not even suspect the existence. Like Israel of old they question, "If God is leading us, why do all these things come upon us?"

These things come upon them because God is leading them. Trials and obstacles are the Lord's chosen methods of discipline and His appointed conditions of success. He who reads human hearts knows the character better than people know themselves. He sees that some have powers and susceptibilities that, rightly directed, might be used in the advancement of His work. In His providence He brings these persons into different positions and varied circumstances that they may discover in their character the defects that have been concealed from their own knowledge. He gives them opportunity to correct these defects and to fit themselves for His service. Often He permits the fires of affliction to assail them that they may be purified.

The fact that we are called upon to endure trial shows that the Lord Jesus sees in us something precious that He desires to develop. If He saw in us nothing whereby He might glorify His name, He would not spend time refining us. He does not cast worthless stones into His furnace; it is valuable ore that He refines. The blacksmith puts the iron and steel into the fire that he may know what manner of metal they are. The Lord allows His chosen ones to be placed in the furnace of affliction to prove their mettle and whether they can be fashioned for His work.

The potter takes the clay and molds it according to his will. He kneads it and works it. He tears it apart and presses it together. He wets it and then dries it. He lets it lie for a while without touching it. When it is perfectly pliable, he continues the work of making it into a vessel. He forms it into shape and on the wheel trims and polishes it. He dries it in the sun and bakes it in the oven. Thus it becomes a vessel fit for use. So the great Master Worker desires to mold and fashion us. And as the clay is in the hands of the potter, so we are to be in His hands. We are not to try to do the work of the potter. Our part is to yield ourselves to be molded by the Master Worker.

"Beloved, do not think it strange concerning the fiery trial which is to try you, as though some strange thing happened to you; but rejoice to the extent that you partake of Christ's sufferings, that when His glory is revealed, you may also be glad with exceeding joy." 1 Peter 4:12, 13.

In the full light of day, and hearing the music of other voices, the caged bird will not sing the song that his master seeks to teach him. He learns a snatch of this, a trill of that, but never a separate and entire melody. But the master covers the cage and places it where the bird will listen to the one song he is to sing. In the dark he tries and tries again to sing that song until it is learned, and he breaks forth in perfect melody. Then the bird is brought out, and ever afterward he can sing that song in the light. Thus God deals with His children. He has a song to teach us, and when we have learned it amid the shadows of affliction we can sing it ever afterward.

Many are dissatisfied with their lifework. It may be that their surroundings are uncongenial. Or perhaps their time is occupied with commonplace work when they think themselves capable of higher responsibilities. Often their efforts seem to them to be unappreciated or fruitless. Their future is uncertain.

Let us remember that while the work we have to do may not be our choice, it is to be accepted as God's choice for us. Whether pleasing or unpleasing, we are to do the duty that lies nearest. "Whatever your hand finds to do, do it with your might; for there is no work or device or knowledge or wisdom in the grave where you are going." Ecclesiastes 9:10. If the Lord desires us to bear a message to Nineveh, it will not be as pleasing to Him for us to go to Joppa or Capernaum. He has reasons for sending us to the place toward which we have been directed. At that very place there may be someone in need of the help we can give. He who sent Philip to the Ethiopian councilor, Peter to the Roman centurion, and the little Israelite maiden to the help of Naaman, the Syrian captain, sends men and women and youth today as His representatives to those in need of divine help and guidance.

God's Plans Are Best

Our plans are not always God's plans. He may see that it is best for us and for His cause to refuse our very best intentions, as He did when King David wanted to build the temple. But of one thing we may be assured, He will bless and use in the advancement of His cause those who sincerely devote themselves and all they have to His glory. If He sees it best not to grant their desires, He will counterbalance the refusal by giving them tokens of His love and entrusting to them another service.

In His loving care and interest for us, often He who understands us better than we understand ourselves refuses to permit us selfishly to seek the gratification of our own ambition. He does not permit us to pass by the simple but sacred duties that lie near us. Often these duties afford the very training essential to prepare us for a higher work. Often our plans fail that God's plans for us may succeed.

We are never called upon to make a real sacrifice for God. He asks us to yield many things to Him, but in doing this we are only giving up that which hinders us in the heavenward way. Even when called upon to surrender those things that in themselves are good, we may be sure that God is working out for us some higher good.

In the future life the mysteries that here have annoyed and disappointed us will be made plain. We shall see that our seemingly unanswered prayers and disappointed hopes have been among our greatest blessings.

We are to look upon every duty, however humble, as sacred because it is a part of God's service. Our daily prayer should be, "Lord, help me to do my best. Teach me how to do better work. Give me energy and cheerfulness. Help me to bring into my service the loving ministry of the Savior."

A Lesson From the Life of Moses

Consider the experience of Moses. The education he received in Egypt as the king's grandson and prospective heir to the throne was very thorough. Nothing was neglected that was calculated to make him a wise man, as the Egyptians understood wisdom. He received the highest civil and military training. He felt that he was fully prepared for the work of delivering Israel from bondage. But God judged otherwise. His providence appointed Moses forty years of training in the wilderness as a keeper of sheep.

The education that Moses had received in Egypt was a help to him in many respects, but the most valuable preparation for his lifework was that which he received while employed as a shepherd. Moses was naturally of an impetuous spirit. In Egypt, as a successful military leader and favorite with the king and the nation, he had been accustomed to receiving praise and flattery. He had attracted the people to himself. He hoped to accomplish by his own powers the work of delivering Israel.

Far different were the lessons he had to learn as God's representative. As he led his flocks through the wilds of the mountains and into the green pastures of the valleys, he learned faith and meekness, patience, humility, and self-forgetfulness. He learned to care for the weak, to nurse the sick, to seek after the straying, to bear with the unruly, to tend the lambs, and to nurture the old and feeble.

In this work Moses was drawn nearer to the Chief Shepherd. He became closely united to the Holy One of Israel. No longer did he plan to do a great work. He sought to do faithfully as unto God the work committed to his charge. He recognized the presence of God in his surroundings. All nature spoke to him of the Unseen One. He knew God as a personal God, and in meditating upon His character he grasped more and more fully the sense of His presence. He found refuge in the everlasting arms.

After this experience Moses heard the call from heaven to exchange his shepherd's staff for the rod of authority, to leave his flock of sheep and take the leadership of Israel. The divine command found him self-distrustful, slow of speech, and timid. He was overwhelmed with a sense of being incapable of being a mouthpiece for God. But he accepted the work, putting his whole trust in the Lord. The greatness of his mission called into exercise the best powers of his mind. God blessed his ready obedience, and he became eloquent, hopeful, self-possessed, fitted for the greatest work ever given to man. Of him it is written: "Since then there has not arisen in Israel a prophet like Moses, whom the Lord knew face to face." Deuteronomy 34:10.

Let those who feel that their work is not appreciated and who crave a position of greater responsibility consider that "exaltation comes neither from the east nor from the west nor from the south. But God is the Judge: He puts down one, and exalts another." Psalm 75:6, 7. Every person has a place in the eternal plan of heaven. Whether we fill that place depends upon our own faithfulness in cooperating with God.

We need to beware of self-pity. Never indulge the feeling that you are not esteemed as you should be, that your efforts are not appreciated, that your work is too difficult. Let the memory of what Christ endured for us silence every murmuring thought. We are treated better than was our Lord. "'Do you seek great things for yourself? Do not seek them.'" Jeremiah 45:5. The Lord has no place in His work for those who have a greater desire to win the crown than to bear the cross. He wants people who are more intent upon doing their duty than upon receiving their reward—men and women who are more concerned for principle than for promotion.

Those who are humble and who do their work as unto God may not make as great a show as do those who are full of bustle and self-importance, but their work counts for more. Often those who make a great parade call attention to self, interposing between the people and God, and their work proves a failure. "'Wisdom is the principal thing; therefore get wisdom. And in all your getting, get understanding. Exalt her, and she will promote you; she will bring you honor, when you embrace her.'" Proverbs 4:7, 8.

Many become stereotyped in a wrong course of action because they have not the determination to take themselves in hand and reform. But this need not be. They may cultivate their powers to do the very best kind of service, and then they will always be in demand. They will be valued for all that they are worth.

If any are qualified for a higher position, the Lord will lay the burden not on them alone but on those who have tested them, who know their worth, and who can understandingly urge them forward. Those who perform their appointed work faithfully day by day will in God's own time hear His call, "Come up higher."

While the shepherds were watching their flocks on the hills of Bethlehem, angels from heaven visited them. So today while humble workers for God are following their employment, angels of God stand by their side, listening to their words and noting the manner in which their work is done, to see if larger responsibilities may be entrusted to them.

God does not estimate people by their wealth, their education, or their position. He estimates them by their purity of motive and beauty of character. He looks to see how much of His Spirit they possess and how much of His likeness their life reveals. To be great in God's kingdom is to be as a little child in humility, in simplicity of faith, and in purity of love.

"'You know,'" Christ said, "'that the rulers of the Gentiles lord it over them, and those who are great exercise authority over them. Yet it shall not be so among you; but whoever desires to become great among you, let him be your servant.'" Matthew 20:25, 26.

Of all the gifts that heaven can bestow upon human beings, fellowship with Christ in His sufferings is the most weighty trust and the highest honor. Not Enoch, who was translated to heaven, not Elijah, who ascended in a chariot of fire, was greater or more honored than John the Baptist, who perished alone in a dungeon. "To you it has been granted on behalf of Christ, not only to believe in Him, but also to suffer for His sake." Philippians 1:29.

Plans for the Future

Many are unable to make definite plans for the future. Their life is unsettled. They cannot see exactly how matters will develop, and this often fills them with anxiety and unrest. Let us remember that the life of God's children in this world is a pilgrim life. We have not wisdom to plan our own lives. It is not for us to shape our future. "By faith Abraham obeyed when he was called to go out to the place which he would receive as an inheritance. And he went out, not knowing where he was going." Hebrews 11:8.

Christ in His life on earth made no plans for Himself. He accepted God's plans for Him, and day by day the Father unfolded His plans. So should we depend upon God, that our lives may be the simple outworking of His will. As we commit our ways to Him, He will direct our steps.

Too many, in planning for a brilliant future, make an utter failure. Let God plan for you. As a little child, trust to the guidance of Him who will "'guard the feet of His saints.'" 1 Samuel 2:9. God never leads His children otherwise than they would choose to be led if they could see the end from the beginning and discern the glory of the purpose that they are fulfilling as co-workers with Him.

Wages

When Christ called His disciples to follow Him, He offered them no flattering prospects in this life. He gave them no promise of gain or worldly honor, nor did they stipulate what they should receive. To Matthew as he sat collecting taxes, the Savior said, "'Follow Me.' And he left all, rose up, and followed Him." Luke 5:27, 28. Before giving service, Matthew did not wait to demand a certain salary equal to the amount received in his former occupation. Without question or hesitation he followed Jesus. It was enough for him that he was to be with the Savior, that he might hear His words and unite with Him in His work.

So it was with the disciples called previously. When Jesus invited Peter and his companions to follow Him, immediately they left their boats and nets. Some of these disciples had friends dependent on them for support, but when they received the Savior's invitation they did not hesitate and inquire, "How shall I live and sustain my family?" They were obedient to the call, and when Jesus asked them later, "'When I sent you without money bag, sack, and sandals, did you lack anything?'" they could answer, "'Nothing.'" Luke 22:35.

Today the Savior calls us to His work as He called Matthew and John and Peter. If our hearts are touched by His love, the question of compensation will not be uppermost in our minds. We shall rejoice to be co-workers with Christ, and we shall not fear to trust His care. If we make God our strength, we shall have clear perceptions of duty and unselfish aspirations. Our life will be actuated by a noble purpose that will raise us above selfish, unworthy motives.

God Will Provide

Many who profess to be Christ's followers have an anxious, troubled heart because they are afraid to trust themselves with God. They do not make a complete surrender to Him, for they shrink from the consequences that such a surrender may involve. But unless they do make this surrender, they cannot find peace.

There are many whose hearts are aching under a load of care because they seek to reach the world's standard. They have chosen its service, accepted its perplexities, adopted its customs. Thus their character is marred and their life made a weariness. Continual worry is wearing out their life forces. Our Lord desires them to lay aside this yoke of bondage. He invites them to accept His yoke. He says, "'My yoke is easy and My burden is light.'" Worry is blind and cannot discern the future, but Jesus sees the end from the beginning. In every difficulty He has His way prepared to bring relief. "No good thing will He withhold from those who walk uprightly." Matthew 11:30; Psalm 84:11.

Our heavenly Father has a thousand ways to provide for us of which we know nothing. Those who accept the one principle of making the service of God supreme will find perplexities vanish and a plain path before their feet.

The faithful discharge of today's duties is the best preparation for tomorrow's trials. Do not gather together all tomorrow's liabilities and cares and add them to the burden of today. "'Sufficient for the day is its own trouble.'" Matthew 6:34.

Let us be hopeful and courageous. Despondency in God's service is sinful and unreasonable. He knows our every necessity. Our covenant-keeping God unites the gentleness and care of the tender shepherd with the omnipotence of the King of kings. His power is absolute, and it is the pledge of the sure fulfillment of His promises to all who trust in Him. He has means for the removal of every difficulty, that those who serve Him and respect the means He employs may be sustained. His love is as far above all other love as the heavens are far above the earth. He watches over His children with a love that is measureless and everlasting.

In the darkest days, when appearances seem most forbidding, have faith in God. He is working out His will, doing all things well in behalf of His people. The strength of those who love and serve Him will be renewed day by day.

He is able and willing to bestow upon His servants all the help they need. He will give them the wisdom that their varied necessities demand. Said the tested and faithful apostle Paul: "He said to me, 'My grace is sufficient for you, for My strength is made perfect in weakness.' Therefore most gladly I will rather boast in my infirmities, that the power of Christ may rest upon me. Therefore I take pleasure in infirmities, in reproaches, in needs, in persecutions, in distresses, for Christ's sake. For when I am weak, then I am strong." 2 Corinthians 12:9, 10.

C h a p t e r   4 1

In Contact
With Others

Every association of life calls for the exercise of self-control, forbearance, and sympathy. We differ so widely in disposition, habits, and education that our ways of looking at things vary. We judge differently. Our understanding of truth, our ideas in regard to the conduct of life, are not in all respects the same. The experience of no two people is alike in every particular. The trials of one are not the trials of another. The duties that one finds light are to another most difficult and perplexing.

So frail, so ignorant, so liable to misconception is human nature, that all of us should be careful in the estimate we place upon another. We little know the bearing of our acts upon the experience of others. What we do or say may seem to us of little consequence, but if our eyes could be opened, we would see that upon it depended the most important results for good or for evil.

Consideration for Burden Bearers

Many have carried so few burdens, their hearts have known so little real anguish, and they have felt so little perplexity and distress in behalf of others, that they cannot understand the work of true burden bearers. They are no more capable of appreciating the heavy responsibilities that others carry than are children of understanding the care and toil of their burdened father. Children may wonder at their father's fears and perplexities. These appear needless to them. But when years of experience have been added to their lives, when they themselves come to bear heavy burdens, they will look back upon their father's life and understand that which once was so incomprehensible. Bitter experience has given them knowledge.

The work of many burden bearers is not understood or appreciated until death lays them low. When others take up the burdens they have laid down and meet the difficulties they encountered, then associates can understand how faith and courage were tested. Often the mistakes they were so quick to censure are lost sight of. Experience teaches them sympathy. God permits men and women to be placed in positions of responsibility. When they err, He has power to correct or to remove them. We should be careful not to take into our hands the work of judging that belongs to God.

The conduct of David toward Saul has a lesson. By command of God, Saul had been anointed king over Israel. Because of his disobedience the Lord declared that the kingdom should be taken from him, and yet how tender and courteous and forbearing was the conduct of David toward him! In attempting to find David and kill him, Saul came into the wilderness and, unattended, entered the very cave where David with his men of war lay hidden.

"Then the men of David said to him, 'This is the day of which the Lord said to you, . . . "I will deliver your enemy into your hand, that you may do to him as it seems good to you."' . . . And he said to his men, 'The Lord forbid that I should do this thing to my master, the Lord's anointed, to stretch out my hand against him, seeing he is the anointed of the Lord.'" 1 Samuel 24:4-6.

The Savior bids us, "'Judge not, that you be not judged. For with what judgment you judge, you will be judged; and with the measure you use, it will be measured back to you.'" Remember that soon your life record will pass in review before God. Remember, too, that He has said, "You are inexcusable, O man, whoever you are who judge, . . . for you who judge practice the same things." Matthew 7:1, 2; Romans 2:1.

Forbearance Under Wrong

We cannot afford to let our spirits chafe over any real or supposed wrong done to ourselves. Self is the enemy we most need to fear. No form of vice has a more damaging effect upon the character than has human passion not under the control of the Holy Spirit. No other victory we can gain will be so precious as the victory gained over self.

We should not allow our feelings to be easily wounded. We are to live to save souls, not to guard our feelings or our reputation. As we become interested in the salvation of souls we cease to mind the little differences that so often arise in our association with one another. Whatever others may think of us or do to us, it need not disturb our oneness with Christ, the fellowship of the Spirit. "What credit is it if, when you are beaten for your faults, you take it patiently? But when you do good and suffer, if you take it patiently, this is commendable before God." 1 Peter 2:20.

Do not retaliate. So far as you can do so, remove all cause for misunderstanding. Avoid the appearance of evil. Without sacrificing principle, do all in your power to settle peacefully your differences with others. "'If you bring your gift to the altar, and there remember that your brother has something against you, leave your gift there before the altar, and go your way. First be reconciled to your brother, and then come and offer your gift.'" Matthew 5:23, 24.

If impatient words are spoken to you, never reply in the same spirit. Remember that "a soft answer turns away wrath." Proverbs 15:1. And there is wonderful power in silence. Words spoken in reply to one who is angry sometimes serve only to exasperate. But anger met with silence, in a tender, forbearing spirit, quickly dies away.

Under a storm of stinging, faultfinding words, keep your mind stayed upon the Word of God. Let mind and heart be stored with God's promises. If you are ill-treated or wrongfully accused, instead of returning an angry answer, repeat to yourself precious promises, such as these:

"Do not be overcome by evil, but overcome evil with good." Romans 12:21.

"Commit your way to the Lord, trust also in Him, and He shall bring it to pass. He shall bring forth your righteousness as the light, and your justice as the noonday." Psalm 37:5, 6.

"'There is nothing covered that will not be revealed, nor hidden that will not be known.'" Luke 12:2.

"You have caused men to ride over our heads; we went through fire and through water; but You brought us out to rich fulfillment." Psalm 66:12.

We are prone to look to our associates and other humans for sympathy and uplifting, instead of looking to Jesus. In His mercy and faithfulness God often permits those in whom we place confidence to fail us, in order that we may learn what a mistake it is to make flesh our strength (Jeremiah 17:5). Let us trust fully, humbly, unselfishly in God. He knows the sorrows that we feel to the depths of our being but that we cannot express. When all things seem dark and unexplainable, remember the words of Christ, "'What I am doing you do not understand now, but you will know after this.'" John 13:7.

Study the history of Joseph and of Daniel. The Lord did not prevent the plottings of men who sought to do them harm, but He caused all these devices to work for good to His servants who in the midst of trial and conflict preserved their faith and loyalty.

As long as we are in this world, we shall meet with adverse influences. There will be provocations to test the temper, and by meeting these in a right spirit the Christian graces will develop. If Christ lives in us, we shall be patient, kind, and forbearing, cheerful amid frets and irritations. Day by day and year by year we shall conquer self and grow into a noble heroism. This is our allotted task, but it cannot be accomplished without help from Jesus, resolute decision, unwavering purpose, continual watchfulness, and unceasing prayer. Each one has a personal battle to fight. Not even God can make our characters noble or our lives useful unless we become co-workers with Him. Those who decline the struggle lose the strength and joy of victory.

We do not need to keep our own record of trials, difficulties, griefs, and sorrows. All these things are written in heaven's books, and God will take care of them. While we are counting up the disagreeable things, many things that are pleasant to reflect upon pass from memory, such as the merciful kindness of God surrounding us every moment, and the love over which angels marvel, that God gave His Son to die for us. If as a worker for Christ you feel you have had greater cares and trials than others have had, remember that for you there is a peace unknown to those who shun these burdens. There is comfort and joy in the service of Christ. Let the world see that life with Him is no failure.

Think Positive Thoughts

If you do not feel lighthearted and joyous, do not talk of your feelings. Cast no shadow upon the lives of others. A cold, sunless religion never draws souls to Christ. It drives them away from Him into the nets that Satan has spread for the feet of the straying. Instead of thinking of your discouragements, think of the power you can claim in Christ's name. Let your imagination take hold upon things unseen. Let your thoughts be directed to the evidences of the great love of God for you. Faith can endure trial, resist temptation, bear up under disappointment. Jesus lives as our advocate. All is ours that His mediation secures.

Christ values those who live wholly for Him. He visits those who, like the beloved John in exile, are for His sake in hard and trying places. God will not suffer one of His truehearted workers to be left alone, to struggle against great odds and be overcome. He preserves as a precious jewel everyone whose life is hid with Christ in Him. Of every such one He says: "'I . . . will make you like a signet ring; for I have chosen you.'" Haggai 2:23.

Then talk of the promises. Talk of Jesus' willingness to bless. He does not forget us for one brief moment. When, despite disagreeable circumstances, we rest confidingly in His love and shut ourselves in with Him, the sense of His presence will inspire a deep, tranquil joy. Of Himself Christ said: "'I do nothing of Myself; but as My Father taught Me, I speak these things. And He who sent Me is with Me. The Father has not left Me alone, for I always do those things that please Him.'" John 8:28, 29.

The Father's presence encircled Christ, and nothing befell Him but that which infinite love permitted for the blessing of the world. Here was His source of comfort, and it is for us. Those who are imbued with the Spirit of Christ abide in Christ. Whatever comes to them comes from the Savior, who surrounds them with His presence. Nothing can touch them except by the Lord's permission. All our sufferings and sorrows, all our temptations and trials, all our sadness and griefs, all our persecutions and privations—in short, all things—work together for our good. All experiences and circumstances are God's workmen whereby good is brought to us.

If we have a sense of the longsuffering of God toward us, we shall not be found judging or accusing others. When Christ was living on the earth, how surprised His associates would have been if, after becoming acquainted with Him, they had heard Him speak one word of accusation, of fault-finding, or of impatience. Let us never forget that those who love Him are to represent Him in character.

"Be kindly affectionate to one another with brotherly love, in honor giving preference to one another." "Not returning evil for evil or reviling for reviling, but on the contrary blessing, knowing that you were called to this, that you may inherit a blessing." Romans 12:10; 1 Peter 3:9.

Reveal the Christian Graces

The Lord Jesus demands our acknowledgment of the rights of every person. People's social rights, and their rights as Christians, are to be taken into consideration. All are to be treated with refinement and delicacy, as the sons and daughters of God.

Christianity will make a man a gentleman and a woman a lady. Christ was courteous, even to His persecutors, and His true followers will manifest the same spirit. Look at Paul when brought before rulers. His speech before Agrippa is an illustration of true courtesy as well as persuasive eloquence. The gospel does not encourage the formal politeness current with the world, but the courtesy that springs from real kindness of heart.

The most careful cultivation of the outward proprieties of life is not sufficient to shut out all fretfulness, harsh judgment, and unbecoming speech. True refinement will never be revealed so long as self is considered as the supreme object. Love must dwell in the heart. Thoroughgoing Christians draw their motives of action from a deep heart-love for their Master. Up through the roots of their affection for Christ springs an unselfish interest in others. Love imparts to its possessor grace, propriety, and beauty of deportment. It illuminates the countenance and subdues the voice. It refines and elevates the whole being.

Life is chiefly made up of little things, not of great sacrifices and wonderful achievements. Often through the little things that seem unworthy of notice, great good or evil is brought into our lives. Through our failure to endure the tests that come to us in little things, the habits are molded, the character misshaped; and when the greater tests come, they find us unready. Only by acting on principle in the tests of daily life can we acquire power to stand firm and faithful in the most dangerous and difficult positions.

We are never alone. Whether we choose Him or not, we have a companion. Remember that wherever you are, whatever you do, God is there. Nothing that is said or done or thought escapes His attention. To your every word or deed you have a witness—the holy, sin-hating God. Before you speak or act, always think of this. As a Christian, you are a member of the royal family, a child of the heavenly King. Say no word, do no act, that shall bring dishonor on "that noble name by which you are called." James 2:7.

Study carefully the divine-human character, and constantly inquire, "What would Jesus do were He in my place?" This should be the measurement of our duty. Do not place yourself needlessly in the society of those who by their arts would weaken your purpose to do right or lead you to bring a stain upon your conscience. Do nothing among strangers, whether in the street or in the home, that would have the least appearance of evil. Do something every day to improve, beautify, and ennoble the life that Christ has purchased with His own blood.

Always act from principle, never from impulse. Temper the natural impetuosity of your nature with meekness and gentleness. Indulge in no lightness or trifling. Let no low witticism escape your lips. Even the thoughts must not be allowed to run riot. They must be restrained, brought into captivity to the obedience of Christ. Let them be placed upon holy things. Then, through the grace of Christ, they will be pure and true.

We need a constant sense of the ennobling power of pure thoughts. The only security for any soul is right thinking. As a person "thinks in his heart, so is he." Proverbs 23:7. The power of self-restraint strengthens by exercise. That which at first seems difficult, by constant repetition grows easy, until right thoughts and actions become habitual. If we will, we may turn away from all that is cheap and inferior, and rise to a high standard. We may be respected by others and beloved of God.

Speak Well of Others

Cultivate the habit of speaking well of others. Dwell upon the good qualities of those with whom you associate, and see as little as possible of their errors and failings. When tempted to complain of what someone has said or done, praise something in that person's life or character. Cultivate thankfulness. Praise God for His wonderful love in giving Christ to die for us. It never pays to think of our grievances. God calls upon us to think of His mercy and His matchless love, that we may be inspired with praise.

Earnest workers have no time to dwell on the faults of others. We cannot afford to live on the husks of others' faults or failings. Evilspeaking is a twofold curse, falling more heavily upon the speaker than upon the hearer. Those who scatter seeds of dissension and strife reap in their own souls the deadly fruits. The very act of looking for evil in others develops evil in those who do the looking. By dwelling upon the faults of others, we are changed into the same image. But by beholding Jesus, talking of His love and perfection of character, we become changed into His image. By contemplating the lofty ideal He has placed before us, we shall be uplifted into a pure and holy atmosphere, even the presence of God. When we abide here, there goes forth from us a light that brightens and affects all who are connected with us.

Instead of criticizing and condemning others, say, "I must work out my own salvation. If I cooperate with Him who desires to save my soul, I must watch myself diligently. I must put away every evil from my life. I must overcome every fault. I must become a new creature in Christ. Then, instead of weakening those who are striving against evil, I can strengthen them by encouraging words." We are too indifferent in regard to one another. Too often we forget that our associate workers are in need of strength and cheer. Take care to assure them of your interest and sympathy. Help them by your prayers, and let them know that you are praying for them.

Not all who profess to be workers for Christ are true disciples. Among those who bear His name and even are numbered with His workers are some who do not represent Him in character. They are not governed by His principles. These persons are often a cause of perplexity and discouragement to their associates who are young in Christian experience. But none need to be misled. Christ has given us a perfect example. He bids us follow Him.

Till the end of time there will be tares among the wheat. When the servants of the householder, in their zeal for his honor, asked permission to root out the tares, the master said: "'No, lest while you gather up the tares, you also uproot the wheat with them. Let both grow together until the harvest.'" Matthew 13:29, 30.

In His mercy and longsuffering, God bears patiently with the perverse and even the falsehearted. Among Christ's chosen apostles was Judas the traitor. Should we then be surprised or discouraged that there are falsehearted ones among His workers today? If He who reads the heart could bear with him who He knew was to be His betrayer, with what patience should we bear with those at fault.

And not all, even of those who appear most faulty, are like Judas. Peter, impetuous, hasty, and self-confident, often appeared to far greater disadvantage than did Judas. He was reproved more often by the Savior. But what a life of service and sacrifice was his! What a testimony it bears to the power of God's grace! So far as we are capable, we are to be to others what Jesus was to His disciples when He walked and talked with them on earth.

Regard yourself as a missionary, first of all among your co-workers. Often it requires a vast amount of time and labor to win one soul to Christ. And when a soul turns from sin to righteousness, there is joy in the presence of the angels. But are the ministering spirits who watch over these souls pleased to see how indifferently they are treated by some who claim to be Christians? If Jesus dealt with us as we too often deal with one another, who of us could be saved?

Remember, you cannot read hearts. You do not know the motives that prompted the actions that to you look wrong. There are many who have not received a right education. Their characters are warped, they are hard and gnarled, and seem to be crooked in every way. But the grace of Christ can transform them. Never cast them aside, never drive them to discourage-ment or despair by saying, "You have disappointed me, and I will not try to help you." A few words spoken hastily under provocation—just what we think they deserve—may cut the cords of influence that should have bound their hearts to ours.

The consistent life, the patient forbearance, the spirit unruffled under provocation, is always the most conclusive argument and the most solemn appeal. If you have had opportunities and advantages that have not fallen to the lot of others, consider this, and be ever a wise, careful, gentle teacher.

In order to have the wax take a clear, strong impression of the seal, you do not dash the seal upon it in a hasty, violent way. Instead, you carefully place the seal on the soft wax, then quietly, steadily press it down until it hardens in the mold. In like manner deal with human souls. The continuity of Christian influence is the secret of its power, and this depends on how steadfastly you manifest the character of Christ. Help those who have erred, by telling them of your experiences. Show how, when you made grave mistakes, patience, kindness, and helpfulness on the part of others gave you courage and hope.

Until the judgment you will never know the influence of a kind, considerate course toward the inconsistent, the unreasonable, the un-worthy. When we meet with ingratitude and betrayal of sacred trusts, we are roused to show our contempt or indignation. The guilty expect this; they are prepared for it. But kind forbearance takes them by sur-prise and often awakens their better impulses and arouses a longing for a nobler life.

"Brethren, if a man is overtaken in any trespass, you who are spiritual restore such a one in a spirit of gentleness, considering yourself lest you also be tempted. Bear one another's burdens, and so fulfill the law of Christ." Galatians 6:1, 2.

All who profess to be children of God should bear in mind that as missionaries they will be brought into contact with all classes of minds. There are the refined and the coarse, the humble and the proud, the religious and the skeptical, the educated and the ignorant, the rich and the poor. These varied minds cannot be treated alike, yet all need kindness and sympathy. By mutual contact our minds should receive polish and refinement. We are dependent upon one another, closely bound together as part of the human family.

"Heaven forming each on other to depend,
A master or a servant or a friend,
Bids each on other for assistance call,
Till one man's weakness grows the strength of all."

Through social relations Christianity comes into contact with the world. Every man or woman who has received the divine illumination is to shed light on the dark pathway of those who are unacquainted with the better way. Social power, sanctified by the Spirit of Christ, must be improved in bringing souls to the Savior. Christ is not to be hid away in the heart as a coveted treasure, sacred and sweet, to be enjoyed solely by the possessor. We are to have Christ in us as a well of water, springing up into everlasting life, refreshing all who come in contact with us.

C h a p t e r   42

Development
and Service

Christian life is more than many take it to be. It does not consist wholly in gentleness, patience, meekness, and kindliness. These graces are essential, but there is need also of courage, force, energy, and perseverance. The path that Christ marks out is a narrow, self-denying path. To enter that path and press on through difficulties and discouragements requires people who are more than weaklings.

Force of Character

Men and women of stamina are wanted, leaders who will not wait to have their way smoothed and every obstacle removed, leaders who will inspire with fresh zeal the flagging efforts of dispirited workers, leaders whose hearts are warm with Christian love and whose hands are strong to do their Master's work.

Some who engage in missionary service are weak, nerveless, spiritless, easily discouraged. They lack push. They do not have those positive traits of character that give power to do something—the spirit and energy that kindle enthusiasm. Those who would win success must be courageous and hopeful. They should cultivate not only the passive but the active virtues. While they are to give the soft answer that turns away wrath, they must possess the courage of a hero to resist evil. With the charity that endures all things, they need the force of character that will make their influence a positive power.

Some have no firmness of character. Their plans and purposes have no definite form and consistency. They are of little practical use in the world. This weakness, indecision, and inefficiency should be overcome. There is in true Christian character an indomitableness that cannot be molded or subdued by adverse circumstances. We must have moral backbone, an integrity that cannot be flattered, bribed, or terrified.

God wants us to make use of every opportunity for securing a preparation for His work. He expects us to put all our energies into its performance and to keep our hearts alive to its sacredness and its fearful responsibilities.

Many who are qualified to do excellent work accomplish little because they attempt little. Thousands pass through life as if they had no great object for which to live, no high standard to reach. One reason for this is the low estimate that they place upon themselves. Christ paid an infinite price for us, and according to the price paid He desires us to value ourselves.

Do not be satisfied with reaching a low standard. We are not what we might be, or what it is God's will that we should be. God has given us reasoning powers, not to remain inactive or to be perverted to earthly and sordid pursuits, but that they may be developed to the utmost, refined, sanctified, ennobled, and used in advancing the interests of His kingdom.

None should consent to be mere machines, run by another person's mind. God has given us ability to think and to act, and it is by acting with carefulness, looking to Him for wisdom, that you will become capable of bearing burdens. Stand in your God-given personality. Be no other person's shadow. Expect that the Lord will work in and by and through you.

Never think that you have learned enough, and that you may now relax your efforts. The cultivated mind is the measure of a person. Your education should continue throughout your lifetime. Every day you should be learning and putting to practical use the knowledge gained.

Remember, in whatever position you may serve you are revealing motive and developing character. Whatever your work, do it with exactness, with diligence. Overcome the inclination to seek an easy task.

The same spirit and principles that one brings into the daily labor will be brought into the whole life. Those who desire a fixed amount to do and a fixed salary, and who wish to prove an exact fit without the trouble of adaptation or training, are not the ones whom God calls to work in His cause. Those who study how to give as little as possible of their physical, mental, and moral power are not the workers upon whom He can pour out abundant blessings. Their example is contagious. Self-interest is the ruling motive. Those who need to be watched and who work only as every duty is specified to them are not the ones who will be pronounced "good and faithful." Workers are needed who manifest energy, integrity, diligence, those who are willing to do anything that needs to be done.

Many become inefficient because, for fear of failure, they evade responsibilities. Thus they do not gain that education which results from experience, and which reading and study and all the advantages otherwise gained cannot give them.

Human beings can shape circumstances, but circumstances should not be allowed to shape the man or woman. We should seize upon circumstances as instruments by which to work. We are to master them but should not permit them to master us.

Workers of power are those who have been opposed, baffled, and thwarted. By calling their energies into action, the obstacles they meet prove to be positive blessings to them. They gain self-reliance. Conflict and perplexity call for the exercise of trust in God and for that firmness which develops power.

The Example of Christ

Christ gave no stinted service. He did not measure His work by hours. His time, His heart, His soul, His strength were given to service for the benefit of humanity. Through weary days He toiled, and through long nights He bowed in prayer for grace and endurance that He might do a larger work. With strong crying and tears He sent His petitions to heaven that His human nature might be strengthened, that He might be braced to meet the wily foe in all his deceptive workings and be fortified to fulfill His mission of uplifting humanity. To His workers He says, "I have given you an example, that you should do as I have done." John 13:15.

"The love of Christ," said Paul, "constrains us." 2 Corinthians 5:14. This was the actuating principle of his conduct. It was his motive power. If ever his ardor in the path of duty flagged for a moment, one glance at the cross caused him to gird up anew the loins of his mind and press forward in the way of self-denial. In his work for others he relied much upon the manifestation of infinite love in the sacrifice of Christ, with its subduing, constraining power.

How earnest, how touching, was his appeal: "You know the grace of our Lord Jesus Christ, that though He was rich, yet for your sakes He became poor, that you through His poverty might become rich." 2 Corinthians 8:9. You know the height from which He stooped, the depth of humiliation to which He descended. His feet entered upon the path of sacrifice and turned not aside until He had given His life. There was no rest for Him between the throne in heaven and the cross. His love for the human family led Him to welcome every indignity and suffer every abuse.

Paul admonishes us, "Let each of you look out not only for his own interests, but also for the interests of others." He bids us possess the mind "which was also in Christ Jesus, who, being in the form of God, did not consider it robbery to be equal with God, but made Himself of no reputation, taking the form of a servant, and coming in the likeness of men. And being found in appearance as a man, He humbled Himself and became obedient to the point of death, even the death of the cross." Philippians 2:4-8.

Paul was deeply anxious that the humiliation of Christ should be seen and realized. He was convinced that if people could be led to consider the amazing sacrifice made by the Majesty of heaven, selfishness would be banished from their hearts. The apostle lingers over point after point, that we may in some measure comprehend the wonderful condescension of the Savior in behalf of sinners. He directs the mind first to the position that Christ occupied in heaven in the bosom of His Father. He reveals Him afterward as laying aside His glory, voluntarily subjecting Himself to the humbling conditions of human life, assuming the responsibilities of a servant, and becoming obedient unto death—the most ignominious, revolting, agonizing death—death on the cross. Can we contemplate this wonderful manifestation of the love of God without gratitude and love and a deep sense of the fact that we are not our own? Such a Master should not be served from grudging, selfish motives.

You know, says Peter, "that you were not redeemed with corruptible things, like silver or gold." 1 Peter 1:18. Oh, had these been sufficient to purchase our salvation, how easily it might have been accomplished by Him who says, "'The silver is Mine, and the gold is Mine'"! Haggai 2:8. But the sinner could be redeemed only by the precious blood of the Son of God. Those who, failing to appreciate this wonderful sacrifice, withhold themselves from Christ's service, will perish in their selfishness.

Singleness of Purpose

In the life of Christ, everything was made subordinate to His work, the great work of redemption that He came to accomplish. And the same devotion, the same self-denial and sacrifice, the same subjection to the claims of the Word of God, is to be manifest in His disciples.

All who accept Christ as their personal Savior will long for the privilege of serving God. Contemplating what heaven has done for them, their hearts are moved with boundless love and adoring gratitude. They are eager to signalize their gratitude by devoting their abilities to God's service. They long to show their love for Christ and for His purchased possession. They covet toil, hardship, sacrifice.

True workers for God will do their best, because in so doing they can glorify their Master. They will do right in order to honor the requirements of God. They will endeavor to improve all their faculties. They will perform every duty as unto God. Their one desire will be that Christ may receive homage and perfect service.

There is a picture representing a bullock standing between a plow and an altar, with the inscription, "Ready for either"—ready to toil in the furrow or to be offered on the altar of sacrifice. This is the position of the true child of God—willing to go where duty calls, to deny self, to sacrifice for the Redeemer's cause.

C h a p t e r   43

A Higher
Experience

We need constantly a fresh revelation of Christ, a daily experience that harmonizes with His teachings. High and holy attainments are within our reach. Continual progress in knowledge and virtue is God's purpose for us. His law is the echo of His own voice, giving to all the invitation, "Come up higher. Be holy, holier still." Every day we may advance in the perfection of Christian character.

Those who are engaged in service for the Master need an experience much higher, deeper, broader, than many have yet thought of having. Many who are already members of God's great family know little of what it means to behold His glory and to be changed from glory to glory. Many have a twilight perception of Christ's excellence, and their hearts thrill with joy. They long for a fuller, deeper sense of the Savior's love. Let these cherish every desire of the soul after God. The Holy Spirit works with those who will be worked, molds those who will be molded, fashions those who will be fashioned. Give yourselves the culture of spiritual thoughts and holy communings. You have seen merely the first rays of the early dawn of His glory. As you follow on to know the Lord, you will know that "the path of the righteous is as the light of dawn, that shineth more and more unto the perfect day." Proverbs 4:18, RV, margin.

"'These things I have spoken to you,'" said Christ, "'that My joy may remain in you, and that your joy may be full.'" John 15:11.

Ever before Him, Christ saw the result of His mission. His earthly life, so full of toil and self-sacrifice, was cheered by the thought that He would not suffer all this travail for nothing. By giving His life for the life of sinners, He would restore in humanity the image of God. He would lift us up from the dust, reshape the character after the pattern of His own character, and make it beautiful with His own glory.

Christ saw of the travail of His soul and was satisfied. He viewed the expanse of eternity and saw the happiness of those who through His humiliation would receive pardon and everlasting life. He was wounded for their transgressions, bruised for their iniquities. The chastisement of their peace was upon Him, and with His stripes they were healed. (See Isaiah 53:11, 5.) He heard the shout of the redeemed. He heard the ransomed ones singing the song of Moses and the Lamb. Although He must first receive the baptism of blood, although the sins of the world were to weigh upon His innocent soul, although the shadow of an unspeakable woe was upon Him, yet for the joy that was set before Him He chose to endure the cross; He despised the shame.

This joy all His followers are to share. However great and glorious the hereafter will be, not all our reward is to be reserved for the time of final deliverance. Even here we are by faith to enter into the Savior's joy. Like Moses, we are to endure as seeing the Invisible.

Now the church is militant. Now we are confronted with a world in darkness, almost wholly given over to idolatry.

The Joy of the Lord
There were ninety and nine that safely lay
    In the shelter of the fold,
But one was out on the hills away,
    Far, far from the gates of gold—
Away on the mountains wild and bare,
Away from the tender Shepherd's care.

"Lord, Thou hast here Thy ninety and nine;
    Are they not enough for Thee?"
But the Shepherd made answer: "One of Mine
    Has wandered away from Me,
And although the road be rough and steep,
I go to the desert to find My sheep."

But none of the ransomed ever knew
    How deep were the waters crossed,
Nor how dark was the night that the Lord passed through
    Ere He found His sheep that was lost.
Far out in the desert He heard its cry—
Fainting and helpless, and ready to die.

"Lord, whence are these blood drops all the way
    That mark out the mountain's track?"
"They were shed for one who had gone astray,
    Ere the Shepherd could bring him back."
"Lord, why are Thy hands so rent and torn?"
"They were pierced tonight by many a thorn."

But all through the mountains, thunder-riven,
    And up from the rocky steep,
There rose a cry to the gate of heaven,
    "Rejoice, I have found My sheep!"
And the angels sang around the throne,
    "Rejoice, for the Lord brings back His own!"
                    —Elizabeth C. Clephane.

A View of the Future

But the day is coming when the battle will have been fought, the victory won. The will of God is to be done on earth as it is done in heaven. The nations of the saved will know no other law than the law of heaven. All will be a happy, united family, clothed with the garments of praise and thanksgiving—the robe of Christ's righteousness.

All nature, in its surpassing loveliness, will offer to God a tribute of praise and adoration. The world will be bathed in the light of heaven. The light of the moon will be as the light of the sun, and the light of the sun will be sevenfold greater than it is now.

The years will move on in gladness. Over the scene the morning stars will sing together, the sons of God will shout for joy, while God and Christ will unite in proclaiming, "There shall be no more sin, neither shall there be any more death."

These visions of future glory, scenes pictured by the hand of God, should be dear to His children.

Stand on the threshold of eternity and hear the gracious welcome given to those who in this life have cooperated with Christ, regarding it as a privilege and honor to suffer for His sake. With the angels, they cast their crowns at the feet of the Redeemer, exclaiming, "'Worthy is the Lamb who was slain, to receive power and riches and wisdom, and strength and honor and glory and blessing!' . . . 'Honor and glory and power be to Him who sits on the throne, and to the Lamb, forever and ever!'" Revelation 5:12, 13.

There the redeemed ones greet those who directed them to the uplifted Savior. They unite in praising Him who died that human beings might have the life that measures with the life of God. The conflict is over. All tribulation and strife are at an end. Songs of victory fill all heaven as the redeemed stand around the throne of God. All take up the joyful strain, "'Worthy is the Lamb who was slain'" and has redeemed us to God.

"I looked, and behold, a great multitude which no one could number, of all nations, tribes, peoples, and tongues, standing before the throne and before the Lamb, clothed with white robes, with palm branches in their hands, and crying out with a loud voice, saying, 'Salvation belongs to our God who sits on the throne, and to the Lamb!'" Revelation 7:9, 10.

"'These are the ones who come out of the great tribulation, and washed their robes and made them white in the blood of the Lamb. Therefore they are before the throne of God, and serve Him day and night in His temple. And He who sits on the throne will dwell among them. They shall neither hunger anymore nor thirst anymore; the sun shall not strike them, nor any heat; for the Lamb who is in the midst of the throne will shepherd them and lead them to living fountains of waters. And God will wipe away every tear from their eyes.'" "'There shall be no more death, nor sorrow, nor crying; there shall be no more pain, for the former things have passed away.'" Verses 14-17; 21:4.

We need to keep ever before us this vision of things unseen. It is thus that we shall be able to set a right value on the things of eternity and the things of time. It is this that will give us power to influence others for the higher life.

In the Mount With God

"Come up to Me in the mount," God bids us. To Moses, before he could be God's instrument in delivering Israel, was appointed forty years of communion with Him in the mountain solitudes. Before he delivered God's message to Pharaoh, he spoke with the angel in the burning bush. Before receiving God's law as the representative of His people, he was called into the mount and beheld His glory. Before executing justice on the idolaters, he was hidden in the cleft of the rock, and the Lord said, "'I will proclaim the name of the Lord before you,' 'merciful and gracious, longsuffering, and abounding in goodness and truth, . . . by no means clearing the guilty.'" Exodus 33:19; 34:6, 7. Before Moses laid down, with his life, his burden for Israel, God called him to the top of Pisgah and spread out before him the glory of the Promised Land.

Before the disciples went forth on their mission, they were called up into the mount with Jesus. Before the power and glory of Pentecost, came the night of communion with the Savior, the meeting on the mountain in Galilee, the parting scene on Olivet, with the angels' promise, and the days of prayer and communion in the upper chamber.

When preparing for some great trial or some especially important work, Jesus would resort to the solitude of the mountains and spend the night in prayer to His Father. A night of prayer preceded the ordination of the apostles and the Sermon on the Mount, the transfiguration, the agony of the judgment hall and the cross, and the resurrection glory.

The Privilege of Prayer

We too must have times set apart for meditation and prayer and for receiving spiritual refreshing. We do not value the power and efficacy of prayer as we should. Prayer and faith will do what no power on earth can accomplish. We are seldom, in all respects, placed in the same position twice. We continually have new scenes and new trials to pass through, where past experience cannot be a sufficient guide. We must have the continual light that comes from God.

Christ is ever sending messages to those who listen for His voice. On the night of His agony in Gethsemane, the sleeping disciples did not hear the voice of Jesus. They had a dim sense of the angels' presence but lost the power and glory of the scene. Because of their drowsiness and stupor they failed to receive the evidence that would have strengthened their souls for the terrible scenes before them. Thus today the very people who most need divine instruction often fail to receive it, because they do not place themselves in communion with heaven.

The temptations to which we are daily exposed make prayer a necessity. Dangers beset every path. Those who are seeking to rescue others from vice and ruin are especially exposed to temptation. In constant contact with evil, they need a strong hold upon God lest they themselves be corrupted. Short and decisive are the steps that lead people down from high and holy ground to a low level. In a moment decisions may be made that fix one's condition forever. One failure to overcome leaves the soul unguarded. One evil habit, if not firmly resisted, will strengthen into chains of steel, binding the whole person.

The reason why so many are left to themselves in places of temptation is that they do not keep the Lord always before them. When you permit your communion with God to be broken, your defense is departed from you. Not all your good purposes and good intentions will enable you to withstand evil. You must be men and women of prayer. Your petitions must not be faint, occasional, and fitful, but earnest, persevering, and constant.

It is not always necessary to bow on your knees to pray. Cultivate the habit of talking with the Savior when you are alone, when you are walking, and when you are busy with your daily work. Let your heart be continually uplifted in silent petition for help, for light, for strength, for knowledge. Let every breath be a prayer.

The Need for Jesus

As workers for God we must reach people where they are, surrounded with darkness, sunken in vice, and stained with corruption. But as we keep our minds upon Him who is our sun and shield, the evil that surrounds us will not bring one stain on our garments. As we work to save souls who are ready to perish we shall not be put to shame if we make God our trust. Christ in the heart, Christ in the life, this is our safety. The atmosphere of His presence will fill the soul with abhorrence of all that is evil. Our spirit may be so identified with His that in thought and aim we shall be one with Him.

It was through faith and prayer that Jacob, from being a man of feebleness and sin, became a prince with God. It is thus that you may become men and women of high and holy purpose, of noble life, men and women who will not for any consideration be swayed from truth, right, and justice. All are pressed with urgent cares, burdens, and duties, but the more difficult your position and the heavier your burdens, the more you need Jesus.

It is a serious mistake to neglect the public worship of God. The privileges of divine service should not be lightly regarded. Those who attend upon the sick are often unable to avail themselves of these privileges, but they should be careful not to absent themselves needlessly from the house of worship.

In ministering to the sick, more than in any merely secular business, success depends on the spirit of consecration and self-sacrifice with which the work is done. Those who bear responsibilities need to place themselves where they will be deeply impressed by the Spirit of God. You should have as much greater anxiety than do others for the aid of the Holy Spirit and for a knowledge of God as your position of trust is more responsible than that of others.

Nothing is more needed in our work than the practical results of communion with God. We should show by our daily lives that we have peace and rest in the Savior. His peace in the heart will shine forth in the countenance. It will give to the voice a persuasive power. Communion with God will ennoble the character and the life. People will take knowledge of us, as of the first disciples, that we have been with Jesus. This will impart to workers a power that nothing else can give. Of this power they must not allow themselves to be deprived.

We must live a twofold life—a life of thought and action, of silent prayer and earnest work. The strength received through communion with God, united with earnest effort in training the mind to thoughtfulness and caretaking, prepares one for daily duties and keeps the spirit in peace under all circumstances, however trying.

The Divine Counselor

When in trouble, many think they must appeal to some earthly friend, telling him or her their perplexities, and begging for help. Under trying circumstances unbelief fills their hearts, and the way seems dark. And all the time there stands beside them the mighty Counselor of the ages, inviting them to place their confidence in Him. Jesus, the great Burden Bearer, is saying, "Come to Me, and I will give you rest." Shall we turn from Him to uncertain human beings, who are as dependent upon God as we ourselves are?

You may feel the deficiency of your character and the smallness of your ability in comparison with the greatness of the work. But if you had the greatest intellect ever given to a mortal, it would not be sufficient for your work. "'Without Me you can do nothing,'" says our Lord and Savior. John 15:5. The result of all we do rests in the hands of God. Whatever may happen, lay hold upon Him with steady, persevering confidence.

In your business, in companionship for leisure hours, and in alliance for life, let all the associations you form be entered upon with earnest, humble prayer. You will thus show that you honor God, and God will honor you. Pray when you are fainthearted. When you are desponding, close the lips firmly to others; do not shadow their path, but tell everything to Jesus. Reach up your hands for help. In your weakness lay hold of infinite strength. Ask for humility, wisdom, courage, increase of faith, that you may see light in God's light and rejoice in His love.

Consecration and Trust

When we are humble and contrite we stand where God can and will manifest Himself to us. He is well pleased when we urge past mercies and blessings as a reason why He should bestow on us greater blessings. He will more than fulfill the expectations of those who trust fully in Him. The Lord Jesus knows just what His children need, how much divine power we will appropriate for the blessing of humanity; and He bestows upon us all that we will employ in blessing others and ennobling our own souls. We must have less trust in what we ourselves can do, and more trust in what the Lord can do for and through us. You are not engaged in your own work; you are doing the work of God. Surrender your will and way to Him. Hold nothing back. Make not a single compromise with self. Know what it is to be free in Christ.

The mere hearing of sermons Sabbath after Sabbath, the reading of the Bible through and through, or the explanation of it verse by verse, will not benefit us or those who hear us, unless we bring the truths of the Bible into our individual experience. The understanding, the will, the affections, must be yielded to the control of the Word of God. Then through the work of the Holy Spirit the precepts of the Word will become the principles of the life.

As you ask the Lord to help you, honor your Savior by believing that you do receive His blessing. All power, all wisdom, are at our command. We have only to ask.

Walk continually in the light of God. Meditate day and night upon His character. Then you will see His beauty and rejoice in His goodness. Your heart will glow with a sense of His love. You will be uplifted as if borne by everlasting arms. With the power and light that God imparts, you can comprehend more and accomplish more than you ever before thought possible.

"Abide in Me"

Christ bids us, "'Abide in Me, and I in you. As the branch cannot bear fruit of itself, unless it abides in the vine, neither can you, unless you abide in Me. . . . He who abides in Me, and I in him, bears much fruit; for without Me you can do nothing. . . . If you abide in Me, and My words abide in you, you will ask what you desire, and it shall be done for you. By this My Father is glorified, that you bear much fruit; so you will be My disciples. As the Father loved Me, I also have loved you; abide in My love. . . . You did not choose Me, but I chose you and appointed you that you should go and bear fruit, and that your fruit should remain, that whatever you ask the Father in My name He may give you.'" John 15:4-16.

"'Behold, I stand at the door and knock. If anyone hears My voice and opens the door, I will come in to him and dine with him, and he with Me.'" Revelation 3:20.

"'To him who overcomes I will give some of the hidden manna to eat. And I will give him a white stone, and on the stone a new name written which no one knows except him who receives it.'" Revelation 2:17.

"'He who overcomes . . . I will give him the morning star.'" "'I will write on him the name of My God and the name of the city of My God. . . . And I will write on him My new name.'" Verses 26-28; 3:12.

Every person whose trust is in God will be able to say with the apostle Paul, "I can do all things through Christ who strengthens me." Philippians 4:13. Whatever the mistakes or failures of the past, we may, with the help of God, rise above them. With Paul we may say, "This one thing I do, forgetting those things which are behind, and reaching forth unto those things which are before, I press toward the mark for the prize of the high calling of God in Christ Jesus." Philippians 3:13, 14, KJV.